The Promise
Fat Loss & Fitness System

Your guide to losing body fat forever

⌘

Derek Alessi
Don Alessi Jr.

First Edition
Clarence Bros. Press, Inc.
Williamsville, New York

The Promise Fat Loss & Fitness System
Derek Alessi and Don Alessi, Jr.

Published by:
        Clarence Bros. Press, Inc.
        7662 Transit Road
        Williamsville, NY 14221
        www.AlessiFit.com

Cover design by Dunn & Associates Design
Interior design and layout by Lee Lewis, Words+Design, 888-883-8347
Back cover copy by Susan Kendrick Writing

Printed in the United States of America

Library of Congress Control Number: 2001119896

ISBN: 0-9705980-0-9

Contents

Foreword   ix

Introduction   1

Part I: The Truth

I.	Never diet again!	7
II.	Let your lean muscle tissue burn your body fat	13
III.	Eat like a Viking!	19
IV.	Burn, baby, burn!	25
V.	Cheating is legal!	31
VI.	All fat is not created equally!	35
VII.	Sugar warning!	39
VIII.	Don't be fooled by slick marketers	47
IX.	Aerobic exercise can make you fatter	57
X.	Spend less time in the gym	63
XI.	Continuing the same workout will result in—nothing!	67
XII.	There is no such thing as the perfect time!	73

Part II: A New Life

XIII.	Begin your transformation	79
XIV.	Questions and answers	89
XV.	Words of encouragement	99

Part III: Time to Eat!

XVI.	Sample meal plans and grocery list	107

Part IV: Body in Motion

XVII.	Exercise instructions	117
XVIII.	The workouts	121
XIX.	A visual guide to the exercises	155
XX.	Chart your progress	171
XXI.	Maintain your success!	191

Glossary   193

Sources of information   197

Dedication

I would like to dedicate this book to all of the wonderful clients with whom I have had the privilege of working to shape their health and fitness over the years. Their trust in my system and me has helped us all to accomplish so much.

I would also like to dedicate this book to all of the well-intentioned individuals who want to improve their health and fitness, but have fallen victim to misleading information. You still have time to transform your life. In this book I will walk you through the transformation, step-by-step, that will improve your life permanently—as long as you stick with it and don't give up!

Acknowledgements

I believe that there is no greater job a person can have than to help enable a dedicated person improve his or her health and fitness. Throughout my career, I have had the great fortune of assisting people to dramatically transform their lives. This endeavor is both challenging and exciting, particularly for those of you who are about to read this book. I know that if you are committed to this program, you will be successful in achieving your goals.

Through the years, I have had help developing this program, as well as writing this book. I would like to acknowledge and thank the individuals who have aided me in this pursuit. They include first and foremost my family:

My brother and business partner, Don. We have battled body fat and helped teach and encourage individuals to take better care of their health and fitness for the past ten years. Don is constantly bettering himself through his tireless research of fitness principles. He was instrumental in developing the workout and exercise section of this system, as well as providing invaluable research. I consider Don the best personal trainer in the business.

My wonderful wife Andrea, who has been with me and supported me through all of the ups and downs; she is and will always be my biggest fan.

My mother and father have also been supportive of Don's and my pursuits in weight training and exercise, even years ago when they thought that we were going to kill ourselves with those weights in the basement!

I would like to thank my editors, Brenda P. Haughey, Ph.D. and Dorothy and Ray Miller. Thanks to them, this book is readable. Bonnie Shiesley and Robert Rivera, personal trainers at Alessi Fitness, also deserve thanks for their assistance with typing the book and gathering the research upon which it is based. Lastly, I would like to thank Robert "Bobby" Corey for his computer knowledge in allowing this book to seamlessly interact with our website.

Disclaimer

The Promise Fat Loss & Fitness System is designed to provide information about increasing your health and fitness. It is solely for informational and educational purposes and is not intended to provide medical advice. You are advised to consult with your physician or health care professional prior to beginning any exercise or nutrition program or if you have any concerns about your health. The Promise Fat Loss & Fitness System is intended for use by healthy individuals eighteen years of age or older. The author, Alessi Fitness Inc., and Clarence Bros. Press Inc. shall have neither liability nor responsibility to any person or entity with respect to any loss, damage or injury alleged to be caused directly or indirectly by the information contained in this system.

Foreword

The Commitment

I congratulate you on your decision to transform your current state of health and fitness. Whether your goal is to shape and tone your body, increase your strength or dramatically reduce your body fat, this system will help you be successful.

It doesn't matter if you are male or female. It doesn't matter if you are eighteen or eighty years old. It doesn't matter if you have ever been in shape before or ever stuck with an organized exercise plan for more than the two weeks after a New Year's resolution. You have the power to *transform* your health and fitness. You have the power to benefit from increased energy and productivity. You have the power to wear clothes that reveal your new shape. And you also have the power to increase your enjoyment of life.

First, let me tell you that I don't intend to waste your valuable time. The information I will be sharing with you is cutting edge technology. The system I propose will work *100 percent* of the time. However, you must first make a commitment to the system. I need you to commit your time and effort to this system exactly as it is presented. This system is just like your education in school (only more exciting!). The more you put into it, the more you'll get out of it. So,

I encourage you *not* to begin this system unless you absolutely commit to:

- Dedicating yourself to improving your health and fitness
- Dedicating yourself to following and completing the system
- Dedicating yourself to becoming the best you have ever been

If you have the discipline and are committed you will succeed—I PROMISE your success!

The Promise

No one intentionally sets out to become fat, out of shape or unhealthy, just as no one sets out to become lonely, bald or broke. It "just happens." The reason it happens is because most people don't have a plan for maintaining and improving their physical selves. While many establish financial or career plans, they do not do so for their health and fitness because they don't perceive it as important.

Hundreds of people have told me they simply don't have the time to dedicate to their health and fitness. They claim they must focus all of their time and energy on their work. I PROMISE if you do not make time for your health and fitness, you won't be able to work toward building your career or material wealth for long. You will either not have the strength and energy to cope with your highly stressful job and will suffer lack of production or, worse yet, you will become like hundreds and thousands of individuals who suffer each year from heart disease, stroke, diabetes (type two is ninety-five percent preventable) and hypertension.

I personally work with many wealthy clients who have neglected their health to build their wealth, and who then attempt to use their wealth to buy back their health. Often they are unsuccessful at reversing the effects of obesity, diabetes, heart disease, osteoporosis and chronic fatigue. Every one of these clients tell me the same thing: "I wish I would have taken better care of my health and fitness sooner." Ironically, they aren't able to enjoy the material wealth they sacrificed their health to attain.

My goal for this system is to educate you so that you know the truth about your health and fitness. I want you to know how your metabolism works and how to increase its effectiveness. I want you to know how certain foods react within your body. I want you to discover how an investment of just three hours—or 1.6 percent of the week—will dramatically improve your health and fitness.

I also want you to learn how to take control of your nutritional habits and not to be deceived by misleading food marketers. I want you to understand the fraud behind fitness claims and radical diets. I intend to teach you the basic tools you will need to empower yourself to take control of your body. Your self-confidence, self-respect and sense of personal control will increase if you adhere 100 percent to The Promise Fat Loss & Fitness System.

No one ever said at the end of his or her life, "I wish I had spent more time at the office." Don't let the enjoyment of life pass you by. I PROMISE you will be well on your way to leading a healthier, happier and more productive life by following my system. Are you ready to begin?

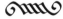

Things do not change; we change.
—Henry David Thoreau

Introduction

Many of my clients over the past ten years have expressed skepticism about beginning a new fitness and weight loss system. These well-intentioned people have paid hard-earned money for weight loss solutions in the past and failed to gain any lasting results. This wasn't because they were unwilling to make the commitment. Rather, it was because the weight loss technology couldn't possibly deliver the benefits it promised.

Many dieters get stuck in what I refer to as the "fly trap." Think of a fly that is stuck inside your car. The fly thinks it can go right through the window, so it rams the window hoping to escape. Then, *wham!* It smashes itself against the window. After taking time to gather its wits, the fly crashes into the window once again, hoping to escape. And *wham!* The fly never learns. It keeps trying the same approach hoping for a different result.

The same thing happens when you go on a diet. You may have tried diets in the past on which you have lost weight initially, but then, *wham!* You still did not achieve the fitness or health results you wanted. Perhaps you even became fatter or more out of shape after the diet. So you tried another diet, hoping for a different outcome. As you have learned by now, the end result of any diet will always be—*wham!* In The Promise Fat Loss & Fitness System, I will show you why you cannot ever achieve lasting results through "dieting."

Perhaps you are similar to hundreds of clients with whom I have worked to transform their health and fitness. Before they begin their life-improving journey, they often ask me the following question: If this system works so well, why isn't everyone in great shape?

The answer is because it takes time and effort and, unfortunately, Americans are entangled in the quick-fix, instant gratification syndrome. They are misled into believing they can have whatever they desire in an instant, without making any sacrifices. Year after year, new *deceptive* products and programs hit the market promising to block fat, shape and tone your abs in three minutes a day, or promising that you can eat whatever fattening foods you want as long as you count the points. The common theme among these products is: it's quick, it's easy and it works like magic!

All of these strategies are intended to do one thing—convince you to believe in them and purchase their product. I don't want to sound negative, but you'll *never* reach the health and fitness level that you want by relying on these deceptive approaches. And it isn't because of you; it's because of them! These products and programs are not designed to produce results, and they will not work. They are designed to sell and make money! Do you think that infomercial companies are looking out for your best interest or theirs?

Pharmaceutical companies spend a fortune getting the Food and Drug Administration (FDA) to approve new "diet drugs" and "fat blockers" so that, as soon as the side effects are exposed to the general public, another product can instantly jump in as the next best seller. Food manufacturers have learned to manipulate labeling laws in order to capitalize on the American desire for better nutrition without delivering a better product. Nutritionists are getting their degrees from schools using textbooks that are sometimes more than twenty-five years old, the majority of which are written by food manufacturers. I've met more overweight and out-of-shape nutritionists and dieticians than in-shape and healthy ones.

Lose 30 pounds in 30 days! You see signs and advertisements like this everywhere. Now, would you be more likely to try a product that offers a thirty-day solution or one like The Promise Fat Loss & Fitness System that offers an eighteen-week solution? Most people want it *now*; they would buy the *thirty-second* solution if one were offered! However, they will always be disappointed and revert back to the same state of being frustrated with their bodies. Eventually, Americans must realize that instant gratification doesn't exist in the quest for better health and fitness, no matter what infomercials say. If a product claims that you can lose weight, develop your abs or live longer and the next words resemble "Quick," "Easy," "Works Like Magic," or "Instantly," you are about to hear a lie.

Each year, an estimated 300,000 deaths in the United States are attributed in part to obesity. This nation is the fattest it has ever been and an increasing percentage of the population is living a sedentary lifestyle. According to Claude Bouchard, author of *Physical Obesity and Activity*, "Sedentarism in overweight or obese persons increases the probability that they will be affected by the common morbidities of excess weight or that they will die prematurely."

Bouchard also elaborates on the consequences of common morbidities: "The current epidemic of obesity in children, adolescents, and young adults will translate later into unprecedented numbers of cases of type two diabetes, hypertension, cardiovascular disease, gallbladder disease, postmenopausal breast cancers, osteoarthritis at the knees, back pain, and physical and mental disabilities."

According to Foreyt and Goodrick's article, "The Ultimate Triumph Of Obesity," an estimated $100 billion is spent in the United States each year as a result of the direct and indirect costs of obesity. These authors predict that by the year 2230, *100 percent* of the adult population in the United States will be obese if the obesity rate continues to grow at the current pace!

It should also be noted that the physical fitness—or lack thereof—in parents greatly affects their children. In fact, R.C. Whitaker, in his paper, "Predicting obesity in young adulthood from childhood and parental obesity," states, "Parental obesity is reported to more than double the risk of adult obesity among both obese and non-obese children under ten years of age. And some of this influence is likely to be due to environmental as well as genetic factors." In other words, parents' health and fitness greatly affects their children's health and fitness.

If achieving good health and fitness were as easy as some advertisers lead us to believe, everyone should be in excellent shape. However, in January 2001, the Centers for Disease Control and Prevention published research documenting that sixty-one percent of Americans are overweight. This statistic is astounding given all of the health and fitness research that has been published, the number of health clubs and personal trainers that are available and the abundance of "healthy" foods on the market. This nation is in serious need of improvement. However, I'm not intending to help the entire nation with The Promise Fat Loss & Fitness System; I'm intending to help you. Follow this system and I PROMISE you will be in the best shape and fitness of your life!

Part I
The Truth

Chapter 1

Never diet again!

Jamie, the dieter

Jamie came to me a few years ago wanting to shape and tone her body. She told me that her weight had gone up and down several times over the past two years. She said that she needed specific exercises to "spot" reduce areas of her body. I asked her what her primary goal was and she told me that she wanted to "lose weight." I asked her what kind of weight: muscle, water or fat? Jamie looked confused. No one had ever asked her this question before. She said, "Of course I want to lose fat. Who would want to lose just water weight?"

Next I asked her what activities she had tried to accomplish her goal. She said that she had joined a weight loss clinic a few years ago. I asked her about her experience with the clinic, and she said it was good. She lost seven pounds in the first ten days by cutting her calories to 1,500 per day.

She mentioned that she hit a minor plateau halfway through her second week of dieting. However, she met with her diet advisor at the clinic (a portly woman), who said it was "normal" to hit a plateau. The advisor then instructed Jamie to restrict her calories to 1,100 a day. She promised Jamie this would "jump start" her results. Jamie told me that she lost another five pounds but soon hit anoth-

7

er plateau. Her advisor then told her she would have to lower her caloric intake to 950 calories a day to get to the next level!

Jamie said that, overall, the diet worked well. She lost more than seventeen pounds, but then she cheated. She craved the junk foods she had given up and she was tired of being hungry all the time. She wanted *more food*. Oddly enough, she was quick to point out that the diet had worked, but *she* failed!

I asked Jamie a simple question: "If initially you were losing weight at 1,500 calories a day, then had to cut down to 1,100 calories a day to lose weight, then eventually cut down to 950 calories, do you think that your metabolism was speeding up or slowing down?" I saw confusion on Jamie's face for a few seconds and then a look of shock. She said, "I must have slowed down my metabolism. Derek, I've heard that people can ruin their metabolism by dieting. Is it true?" I answered, "It is absolutely true."

When you diet by restricting calories, you condition your body to burn less fuel. The weight that you lose is water and lean muscle tissue. Remember, I asked Jamie what kind of weight she wanted to lose, muscle, water or fat. She answered "fat." However, "diets" are a short-term trick designed to lose water and lean muscle tissue. The long-term effect of "dieting" is a gain in body fat and a slower metabolism! And this was not the first time Jamie had dieted. In fact, she had lost and gained weight dozens of times before. Jamie was tired of living this "yo-yo" lifestyle.

My first recommendation to Jamie was to stop yo-yo dieting and hide her scale in the attic. Scale weight doesn't matter! If you develop good lean muscle tissue and are properly hydrated with water you will weigh more on the scale. Does this mean that you have gained fat? No! However, dieting gets rid of valuable lean muscle tissue and water while *retaining body fat!*

Never diet again!

Losing water weight can cause cell dehydration and muscle loss. When cell dehydration occurs, water should be replenished quickly by drinking additional water. However, you cannot afford to lose muscle tissue. The less muscle tissue you have, the less fuel (food) your body will burn. Since muscle is composed of roughly eighty percent water, the loss of water will lead to less muscle tissue. Hence, your metabolism will be slower and you will condition your body to become fatter.

"Dieting" will ruin your metabolism!

Weight loss clinic regimens and various diets deceive you with an old trick: they get you to lose water quickly and thus your "scale weight" will be lower. However, you also lose good, valuable muscle and this is extremely detrimental to your fat-reducing goals.

The decrease in lean muscle tissue makes your body less efficient at processing food. At the end of the diet, you may very well be "lighter" on the scale, but your body fat percentage will likely be the same or higher than it was pre-diet.

I recently conducted a corporate seminar for a Fortune 500 company educating their employees about how to take control of their health and fitness. The room was filled with more than 250 men and women. I began the seminar by asking the group, "How many people, by a show of hands, have ever been on a diet before?" Nearly every hand in the room went up. I then said, "How many people lost weight on the diet?" Once again nearly every hand went up. Next I said, "How many of you who lost weight, kept the weight off for good?" With nearly 250 people who claimed they lost weight on a diet, not one hand went up stating they kept the weight off for good. Lastly, I asked the group, "How many people here are in the best shape of their lives?" Once again, not one hand went up. I congratulated the group on their honesty, adding, "That's the same result as 99.9 percent of all people who ever diet. You never will keep the weight off for good."

Think back to the last time you dieted. You may have lost "scale weight." In fact, you may even remember that your clothes fit better. However, did you feel that your metabolism was moving at a fast rate? Did you have the energy to work and play from dawn to dusk? Did you feel toned or flabby? Did you keep the weight off for good? Dieting is a yo-yo trap that cannot ever bring long term success. Restrict your calories and you will impair your metabolism. I PROMISE!

Throughout my career, I've learned that most people don't like to diet. It isn't a pleasant experience to deprive yourself of food in exchange for the future hope of looking or feeling better. If you have ever dieted before, I'm sure you remember that you literally counted the days until it was over! Most people think of the pain of dieting the way they think of death. In fact, the first three letters in diet spell the word "die." Since dieting is an unpleasant and *ineffective* alternative, I am going to share with you a new technology that will work 100 percent of the time. If you can commit to this lifestyle, you will never have to "diet" again. This is THE PROMISE!

When I ask most people to define metabolism, they usually start off by telling me how they can just look at a piece of cake and gain weight, while a friend or relative of theirs can eat whatever they want and never gain a pound. Let me start by defining metabolism. Metabolism is the rate or speed at which your body processes food. When your metabolism is fast, you will process food quickly. Unless you have a medical condition such as hypothyroidism, or are using certain medications, everyone can increase his or her metabolism.

I know this seems hard to believe, but you can absolutely take control of and choose the rate of your metabolism. You can condition your metabolism to process food at a staggering rate and you can burn more calories and eat more food than you ever dreamed possible. And you can do it without dangerous and expensive over-the-counter "metabolism increasing" drugs, without prescription "fat blockers" and best of all, without ever starving or going on a "diet."

The story about Jamie in the beginning of the chapter, like others I will share with you, is based on actual conversations I have had with my clients over the years. However, their names have been changed to protect their privacy.

I don't blame Jamie—she was a victim of the diet industry. I want to believe that the weight loss clinic did not deceive her intentionally. However, she was victimized by misinformation. No one can ever lose body fat permanently by calorie restriction alone. The *only* way to increase metabolism and lose fat is by 1) developing lean muscle tissue through resistance training 2) increasing the frequency of eating supportive foods and 3) performing a moderate amount of cardiovascular exercise. I call this concept SYNERGY. I teach my personal fitness clients how to use SYNERGY to create the body of their dreams.

The word synergy, by definition, is the combined effect of two or more agents that is greater than the effect of either of the agents used alone. For fitness purposes, I refer to synergy as the combined effect of the development of lean muscle tissue, the frequency of eating supportive meals and a moderate amount of cardiovascular exercise. When weight training and supportive nutrition are performed individually, they have a metabolic effect (increasing metabolism) of ten percent. When cardiovascular exercise is performed alone it has a metabolic effect of five percent. When these components are performed in unison, they have an enormous synergistic metabolic effect of thirty to forty percent! So the best metabolic effect and measurable results will occur when these components are performed together.

This book will teach you how to sensibly incorporate these three synergistic components into your life in order to *transform* your body and improve your health permanently.

Never diet again!

Synergy chart

Activity performed alone	Metabolic increase
Weight training	10%
Supportive nutrition	10%
Cardiovascular exercise	5%
Activities performed together	**30–40%**

Summary

- If you want to reduce your body fat for the rest of your life, *never* diet again.

- Restricting calories or "dieting" will slow down your metabolism.

- When you "diet," you condition your body to burn less fat and fewer calories.

- SYNERGY is the *only* way to permanently increase your metabolism.

- SYNERGY means 1) developing lean muscle tissue 2) increasing the frequency of eating supportive meals and 3) performing a moderate amount of cardiovascular exercise.

Chapter II

 # Let your lean muscle tissue burn your body fat

Karen, the toner

I am fortunate to own a private personal training center across the street from a large health club. One day, Karen came storming into my gym and asked to speak to me about training. I could see that she was agitated about something, but before I could speak she blurted out, "How many treadmills do you have here?" I playfully answered, "How many do you need?" She said that the reason she asked was because she was "sick and tired" of waiting for treadmills at the health club across the street. I asked her, "How often do you walk on the treadmill?" She answered, "Every day for about sixty minutes."

Karen was about thirty-five years old, five feet six inches, and I would estimate about 175 to 180 pounds. She was large for someone who worked out for an hour every day. I asked her to describe her fitness goals. She replied, "I want to shape and tone my body." I then asked her why she walked so much on the treadmill. She said, "I read somewhere that walking is the best exercise you can do for toning the body." I asked her if she had ever done resistance or weight training. She said, "No, I'm big boned and I don't want to get bulky. I just want to *tone*."

I asked Karen how many years she had been doing all this walking. She said, "For about two years." Then I asked her, "How many years do you think it will take to lose the weight you want and tone your body by *just* walking?" She didn't have an answer. I said, "Unfortunately, Karen, it wouldn't happen in 100 years!"

I spent the next hour explaining to Karen that the only way the body burns calories and fat is through lean muscle tissue. If you don't have much lean muscle tissue, you won't burn many calories. I also told her that lean muscle is not big and bulky, *it is lean!* In fact, muscle tissue takes up four times *less* space than fat tissue! I informed her that she didn't have to give up walking on the treadmill entirely, but she needed to incorporate weight training into her workout plan and *reduce* the time she spent walking.

Karen was skeptical at first. This new information was completely different than anything that she had ever heard or read in the tabloids at the checkout aisle before. She told me that everyone at the big health club across the street recommended walking more and doing weight training less. I asked her, "Were the people walking on the treadmill fatter or thinner than the people who were in the weight room?" Karen answered, "Now that I think about it, the people who were in the weight room were much thinner and had more muscle tone than the people who just walked." She added, "Yeah, but can this work for me?" I told her I PROMISE it will work.

That consultation took place more than four years ago. To this day, Karen still trains with me three times a week and her weight is a lean 145 pounds. More important than her scale weight, Karen reduced her body fat twelve percent and lost four dress sizes! She feels better and looks better than when she was in college. Finally, Karen no longer spends sixty minutes at a time on the treadmill. She incorporates weight training, supportive nutrition and a moderate amount of cardiovascular training into a sensible lifestyle. Karen has finally *toned* her body.

Let your lean muscle tissue burn your body fat!

For you to dramatically take control of your health and fitness, it's important for me to share with you the reasons or science behind

Karen's success. The only way to increase the amount of fat or calories your body can burn is by developing your lean muscle tissue through resistance training. I will constantly reiterate this concept throughout the entire book. If you only learn one thing from this book, it will be that your muscle tissue controls your metabolism and decreases your body fat. If you don't have much muscle tissue, you won't be able to burn enough fat. I PROMISE!

Now let's define some common fitness terms. What is a calorie and what does it mean to burn calories? The definition of a calorie is the amount of heat that is necessary to raise one kilogram of water one degree Celsius. What the heck does that have to do with your metabolism? When you burn calories, you're increasing heat production within your body. The only place in the body that produces heat and, consequently, the only place that burns fat or calories is the muscles or, more specifically, the mito-chondria of the muscle.

Weight training is the fastest way to lower your body fat.

The mitochondria are the powerhouses or energy factories of the muscle. They are the components of the muscle that utilize energy and produce heat. If you increase lean muscle tissue, you will also increase mitochondria. Consequently, if you increase your lean muscle tissue, you increase heat production within your body. The process of heat production uses fuel and burns calories.

Resistance or weight training is the most effective way to develop lean muscle tissue. Bouchard, in *Physical Obesity and Activity*, states, "Interventions that increase the quantity of fat free mass [i.e., resistance training] may also increase fat oxidation and therefore be helpful in minimizing the increase in adiposity." In other words, when you increase your fat-free mass (muscle), you will increase the rate at which your body burns fat. Further, Bouchard believes burning fat will decrease adiposity or body fat.

Developing your lean muscle tissue will increase your metabolism.

I consult with many clients like Karen, who initially believe they only need to perform cardiovascular exercise. Most of these individuals are women who want to shape and tone their bodies. When I first meet with them, I explain how their metabolism works. I teach them how muscle tissue uses energy and produces heat. Thus, much more fat is burned with weight training than with cardiovascular exercise.

I encourage clients to try weight training and cut back on cardiovascular training. While most are apprehensive at first, after about four weeks they tell me that their clothes are fitting better. They usually ask, "But how can this be? I'm exercising less than before, but getting in better shape and reducing more body fat." The answer is simple: they allowed their bodies to gain lean muscle tissue.

As the body ages, muscles naturally atrophy, decreasing in size, strength and density. When muscle breaks down, there is less lean muscle tissue in the body. This is why I'm often asked, "How come I'm getting fatter each year? I'm not eating more or differently than in the past." The answer is they have less muscle tissue than years earlier. In fact, after the age of twenty, for both men and women, the body naturally loses seven pounds of lean muscle tissue every ten years or .7 pounds of lean muscle a year. Once women reach menopause, muscle atrophy more than doubles! Their bodies lose upwards of fifteen pounds of muscle every ten years. This leads to loss of bone density and osteoporosis as well as increased body fat and a slower metabolism. Many women over forty-five years of age experience this phenomenon and have gained fat and lost muscle tone at a rapid pace. Is there any question that resistance training is needed?

Metabolism and muscle tissue are strongly related. The more lean muscle tissue you have, the faster your metabolism will be. This doesn't mean that you have to look like a bodybuilder or Zena (the muscle chick) to speed up your metabolism. It simply means that you need more lean muscle tissue than you currently have.

Muscle takes up four times *less* space then fat. For example, a pound of fat takes up about as much space as your clenched fist, whereas a pound of muscle takes up as much space as a silver dollar. So if you are worried that you will get bigger while exercising, you won't if you replace big bulky body fat with lean tight and toned muscle. I PROMISE you will not be disappointed with your results.

Developing lean muscle tissue is the single most important way to increase your metabolism. Muscle tissue in your body burns fat continuously, even when you are eating, watching TV, at work or sleeping. Increased muscle will speed up your resting metabolic rate (the rate at which you burn fuel while not exercising) and help you burn calories and fat twenty-four hours a day. In fact, for every pound of lean muscle tissue you add to your body, your metabolism will burn an extra fifty calories a day! So one added pound of muscle would burn 18,250 additional calories or five pounds of fat weight a year! If you were to add five pounds of lean muscle tissue to your body, you would burn an additional 91,250 calories or twenty-six pounds of fat a year!

For the purposes of this system, the primary benefit of developing lean muscle tissue is permanently increasing your metabolism and burning fat. Other benefits of strength training and developing lean muscle tissue include:

Muscle takes up four times less space than fat!

- Decreased LDL ("bad" cholesterol)
- Increased HDL ("good" cholesterol)

- Increased joint stability
- Improved bone density
- Improved balance
- Additional strength throughout the entire body
- Prevention of low back problems
- Improved glucose metabolism
- Improved posture and flexibility
- Reduction of high blood pressure
- Additional energy

Let your lean muscle tissue burn your body fat!

Summary

- When you develop lean muscle tissue, you produce heat, which has a metabolic effect of burning fat and calories.

- Increase your lean muscle tissue and you increase heat production within your body.

- The more lean muscle tissue you have, the faster your metabolism will work.

- Lean muscle tissue takes up four times less space than fatty tissue.

Chapter III

Eat like a Viking!

Michael, the meal skipper

When Michael called me for a consultation, his primary goal was to lose weight and increase energy. Michael was forty-six years old, five feet ten inches and weighed 220 pounds. Being a very successful attorney, Michael primarily worked behind a desk and performed little physical activity. Michael told me he heard some wonderful things about me helping people drop fat, lose weight and regain their youth. I told him flattery would get him everywhere!

Michael told me that Jerry, a client of mine, referred him to me. He was impressed with how Jerry looked and how he was able to stick to his workouts with me for the past eighteen months. He said that Jerry had explained to him how important it was to do weight training and a moderate amount of cardiovascular training. Michael told me he understood how developing lean muscle tissue would increase his metabolism. He said he wanted to look and feel like a kid again, like Jerry. I said, "Great! It seems that Jerry is a good student and a great motivator." I asked Michael when he was able to begin his workouts and he said, "Tomorrow morning at 9 a.m." I asked him if he were planning on eating breakfast before the workout and he said, "No, I never eat breakfast. I'm not hungry in the morning."

I asked Michael when he usually ate his first meal of the day and he said, "It depends. Sometimes I'm not hungry until dinner." I said, "If you want to speed up your metabolism, lose weight and feel like a kid again, it is important to eat frequently throughout the day." He asked me what "frequently" meant. I told him to eat every three to three and a half hours or five times a day.

Michael asked, "How am I going to do that? I'll gain weight and, besides, I'm not hungry during the day." I said, "You've gained weight just fine eating only once a day! I PROMISE if you eat the way I recommend, you'll lose fat rapidly." He said, "I understand the importance of eating frequently, but I'm just not hungry." I told him the reason he isn't hungry is because his metabolism is not burning fuel (food) efficiently. He isn't eating enough for the body to burn anything.

I also explained that his eating habits have conditioned his body to utilize less fuel, since infrequent meals will train the body to use as little fuel as possible. The body has an innate, fat-storing response to being starved. When the body feels starved, it slows down, burning fewer calories and expending less energy. This is why "dieting" doesn't work.

If you don't frequently nourish your body with supportive foods, your body will go into "starvation mode" and conserve energy and fat. You'll be unable to develop lean muscle tissue and increase your metabolism. Thus, you'll have little energy and a lot of body fat. Michael told me that no one had ever taken the time to explain it to him before. He just thought the less he ate, the less he would weigh. Unfortunately, this is how many individuals are *deceived* by the weight loss industry.

Michael began eating frequently. He has been one of my very best clients for the past three years and has transformed his waist from a hefty size forty to a slim thirty-four. He lowered his scale weight from 220 pounds of fat and jiggle to 185 pounds of ripple. He also increases his self-esteem to the point where he said, "I can now comfortably take my shirt off when I'm doing yard work!"

Eat like a Viking!

I tell many of my clients to "eat like a Viking." I don't mean you have to eat without utensils and stuff globs of fatty meats, cheeses and a drumstick into your mouth with dirty hands while Nordic warriors are fighting to the death. Rather, make sure you are eating supportive foods frequently. You'll be surprised how much food you can actually eat with this system while drastically reducing your body fat. You'll no longer have to resort to eating like a rabbit, consuming only celery, lettuce and carrots. Also, you will *never* have to starve yourself again.

Remember, metabolism is the speed at which your body uses fuel and processes food. Dieting or not eating will cripple your metabolism. If you want your body to get well-conditioned to burning food, it's very important to put food into the fat burning machine frequently. Also, the lean muscle tissue you are diligently working to increase needs small frequent meals to develop.

I know many people are initially afraid of eating frequently. This is because they have dieted before and think the diets have worked, but they have failed. Many of my clients are convinced if they increase meal frequency, they will gain weight. Well, guess what? Initially, they will! However, once they understand why, they will see this as something very positive.

In the last chapter, you learned why muscle is the single most important factor in increasing metabolism and burning fat. However, your bathroom scale cannot differentiate between good muscle weight and water, bone, fat, and internal organs. The scale just lumps them all together and gives you a grand total. Using the scale is an awful indicator of your actual body composition and progress. Please, hide your scale. It will do more harm than good. I PROMISE.

You will lose inches, not "scale weight," during the first month.

When you develop muscle tissue, your scale weight will increase. Does this mean you are fatter? Absolutely not! You'll be leaner! You've heard before that muscle weighs more than fat. In fact, muscle tissue is 2.2 times more dense than fat. In other words, it is more than twice as heavy! I usually tell my clients not to expect to lose any scale weight during the first month of my system. However, you *will* lose fat and inches around your body.

Remember, if you lose weight and that weight is primarily water and muscle, your new lower weight will be short-term and unhealthy. Your objective is to maintain and increase your lean muscle tissue and water while ridding your body of fat. Weight training is the only way to build lean muscle tissue and increase metabolism.

Now, to get back to meal frequency, the food or fuel you put into your body will be either supportive or not supportive of what you are trying to accomplish in the gym. If the body needs more fuel because of the additional muscle, you need to nourish the body with additional supportive fuel. This will increase the metabolic (fat-burning) effect of the muscle and overall metabolism will increase.

With my clients, I use an analogy comparing their metabolism to a fireplace. A fireplace burns fuel and produces heat just like our bodies do. It's easy to understand that if you don't put any logs on the fire, you won't produce any heat. The same is true for the body. If you eat infrequently, your body will not have any calories to burn. Conversely, if you put too many logs on the fire at the same time, you'll douse the flame and it will take a long time to burn through the wood. If you tend to binge eat and consume a lot at one time, you'll douse your metabolism and it will take a long time to burn through food.

Now, follow me and I will get you out of the fire for good! If you frequently put a few logs on the fire and let them burn, you will produce a flame with much heat. If you eat every three to three and a half hours, your body will produce additional heat and the frequent nourishment will support the development of your lean muscle tissue. When you do this in combination with resistance training (which acts like a bigger fireplace) and a moderate amount of cardiovascular exercise (which acts like quick lighter fluid), fat will be incinerated from your body!

The types of food you consume is also very important. I suggest you eat a supportive meal frequently. (By the way, I have scientifically concluded that it's more pleasurable to eat whole foods than to starve on low calorie, tinfoil wrapped diets!) I define a supportive meal as a serving of foods that contain a lean protein source, a slow-releasing carbohydrate (described later in the text) and a vegetable (preferably green). It's that simple! If you eat three meals a day in this supportive manner and eat a snack between breakfast and lunch and between lunch and dinner, you will decrease your body fat rapidly. A snack or meal between your major meals should be smaller in size and calories (more about that later).

I know what you're thinking: you think I'm as crazy as all of the characters on late night infomercials! How can you possibly eat vegetables with every meal? Let me clear up this question and regain your trust. I don't expect you to eat vegetables every morning, although some are great in omelets. I do expect you to eat vegetables at least twice daily. I recommend you eat vegetables with your lunch and always with dinner. I'll elaborate on various types of supportive foods later in the book.

Eat like a Viking!

Summary

- Eat a supportive meal every three to three and a half hours.

- The more frequently you eat, the more conditioned and efficient your body will become at burning food.

- A supportive meal contains a lean protein, a slow-releasing carbohydrate, and a vegetable (preferably green).

Chapter IV

Burn, baby, burn!
The thermal effect of food

Sandra, the calorie counter

Sandra was a doctor who had been working with me for about three months. She had made some wonderful gains lowing her body fat, increasing lean muscle tissue and energy. However, she wanted to bring her body to the next level. She wanted to dramatically lower her body fat and, to use her words, "rip up!"

I congratulated Sandra on her commitment. It's a nice feeling for me to watch people become passionate about their health and fitness. Only three months ago, Sandra had been hesitant about spending any time working out. In fact, when we first met she told me, "You know, I'm a doctor. It's difficult for me to commit to a dedicated program because I get paged for emergencies all the time." I replied, "Sandra, I know that you're busy, and I know that often you don't have control over your schedule. However, I can guarantee if your body is important to you, you'll never regret working with me to improve it." Sandra said, "Okay, I'll give it a try." Now, three months later, she wants to "rip up." I must be a better motivator than I thought!

Sandra asked me, "What will I have to do to rip up?" I replied, "You'll have to continue to weight train three times a week, perform cardiovascular training twenty to thirty minutes five times a week and eat supportive meals every three to three and a half hours." She said, "No problem. But how many calories should I eat?" I said, "Don't count calories. Just make sure that each serving is the size of your clenched fist." For example, a supportive meal is a fist-sized lean protein source, a fist-sized slow-releasing carbohydrate and a fist-sized vegetable.

Sandra asked, "Why should I do that? Calories are calories." I explained to her that a lean protein source is essential to help repair and develop lean muscle tissue, a slow-releasing carbohydrate helps ensure the body has a stable energy supply, and vegetables are a great source of insoluble fiber, which aids in digestion and general health. Sandra said, "Fine, that's all good, but to rip up, *calories* are still all the same."

I told Sandra that different macronutrients, proteins, carbohydrates and fats have different thermal effects, which means each macronutrient needs a different amount of energy for digestion. For example, protein contains the most complex molecular structure, composed of amino acids in clusters of twenty-two. The body must break apart amino acids into di- and tripeptides. Consequently, this requires a lot of energy or calories to digest. Fats, on the other hand, are extremely easy for the body to digest and don't use much energy or calories in digestion. Carbohydrates use more energy than fats, but less than protein.

Sandra was shocked to hear this. She never learned this in medical school. I wanted her to understand clearly that her body burns calories while it digests food. It burns the most calories eating lean protein sources and the least amount eating fatty foods. I wasn't suggesting she only eat protein, however, I wanted her to recognize that protein has the highest thermal effect of any food group.

Maybe you didn't know the reason why, but you instinctively knew that eating 1,000 calories of ice cream or 1,000 calories of lean chicken, brown rice and green beans isn't the same. Even though they are both 1,000 calories, your body will process and utilize them differently. This is another reason why dieting doesn't work. Even if you stay within your caloric intake on the diet, your body will utilize foods differently.

Sandra, still somwhat apprehensive, began to follow my advice. She wasn't disappointed. Within three months, Sandra slashed her body fat another six percent. She dropped three dress sizes and could finally see toned muscles. Her abdominals were defined. Sandra was ripped!

Your fitness goal may be the same as Sandra's, or you may want to only reduce your body fat minimally. While portion size is important, *do not* count calories. It is more important to your results to realize how your body utilizes food sources. Once you understand this concept, you will be on your way to achieving your fitness goals.

Burn, baby, burn!

Perhaps no one has ever taken the time to explain to you that food has a thermal effect. This means that it requires calories or energy to be processed and burned. Some foods require more calories or energy than others to break down and digest. The foods that require the greatest amount of energy to be utilized by the body are proteins. Protein has a thermal effect of twenty to twenty-five percent, which means if you consume 100 calories of protein, the thermal effect will burn twenty to twenty-five calories. The net effect in your body will only be seventy-five to eighty calories.

The thermal effect of carbohydrates is in the middle. While carbohydrates have gained a negative connotation recently thanks to some radical diets on the market, you still need to consume some because they are vital to your health and energy. Complex carbohydrates have a double peptide bond and typically take longer to break down and be released into the body. Examples of complex carbohydrates are pasta, potatoes, and rice.

Alternately, simple carbohydrates have a single peptide bond (you won't be tested on this) so they are broken down and released into the body more rapidly. Examples of simple carbohydrates are table sugar, candy, fruit and honey. I usually recommend eating simple carbohydrates only on "cheat days." I will elaborate more on this later.

Complex carbohydrates have a thermal effect of ten percent. So if you consume 100 calories of what I term a "slow-releasing carbohydrate," such as brown rice, oatmeal or a sweet potato, you'll burn ten calories in the breakdown of these foods. The net result is ninety calories. I'll discuss the difference between slow- and fast-releasing complex carbohydrates in Chapter VII.

Fat has the lowest thermal effect at five percent. If you consume 100 calories of fat, five calories will be burned in the process. That leaves ninety-five calories remaining to either be utilized as energy or stored as body fat. Thus, it is easy to see that there is more to consider than just counting calories or grams of any particular food.

Thermal effect of food

Food	Thermal effect
Protein	20–25%
Carbohydrates	10%
Fats	5%

The following table lists most supportive foods. Included are lean protein sources, slow-releasing carbohydrates and vegetables.

Supportive Foods

Lean proteins	Slow-releasing carbohydrates	Vegetables
Egg whites	Wheat bread	Broccoli
Egg Beaters	Wheat pasta	Spinach
Chicken breast	Sweet potatoes/yams	Green beans
Turkey breast	Oatmeal	Asparagus
Steak	Brown rice	Mushrooms
Fish	Wild rice	Cauliflower
Shellfish	Whole grain couscous	Leafy lettuce
Cottage cheese (1%)		Peppers
Ostrich		
Pork		
Veal		
Buffalo (not the city)		
Tuna		
Protein powders		
Tofu		

Another question clients usually ask is, "How much should I eat at one time?" I doubt that you really want to get into the process of weighing or measuring all of your foods before you eat. The simplest way to ensure you are consuming the appropriate serving size of food is this: each portion should be the size of your clenched fist. For example, a supportive meal would be a fist-sized chicken breast, a fist-sized portion of broccoli and a fist-sized amount of brown rice. If you use your fist as a guide, you will always know how much to eat. Snacks eaten between major meals should be smaller in size and contain fewer calories. Reduce the serving size to approximately one-half clenched fist to satisfy this requirement.

I occasionally work with clients who are vegetarians. The challenge with these clients is to ensure they eat enough lean protein sources. Every one of these individuals I have worked with had a small amount of muscle tissue and high body fat. They usually lack vital amino acids, the building blocks of protein, and the development of muscle tissue is difficult at best without adequate protein for the recuperation and repair of muscle tissue (discussed more fully in Chapter XII.).

If you are a vegetarian for religious or ethical reasons I'm

Egg whites are an excellent source of lean protein.

not asking you to alter your commitment. However, if you are a vegetarian because you believe it is a "healthier" way to eat, I encourage you to re-examine your eating practices. I don't believe having a lack of protein and essential amino acids, high body fat and a low amount of lean muscle tissue is necessarily healthier. According to Joyce Forte in her article, "Vegetarians Versus Meat Eaters," "Vegetarians overall run a high risk of incomplete nutrition, but vegans (no meat, eggs, diary, gelatin or honey) run the highest risk of incomplete nutrition as important vitamins and minerals are omitted from their diets."

If you are a vegetarian and willing to drink protein powders (see Chapter XIII), it's possible for you to consume an adequate amount of protein. This will help with the development of lean muscle tissue and the reduction of body fat without eating animal products. If you are unwilling to consume protein powders, your development of muscle tissue will be difficult at best and your body fat will remain high. Remember, protein contains vital amino acids, vitamins and minerals your body needs to function properly.

Burn, baby, burn!

Summary

- Fats are high in calories and have little thermal effect.

- Compared to fats, complex carbohydrates are lower in calories, provide useful energy and have a greater thermal effect.

- Proteins are essential and provide twice as much thermal effect as carbohydrates or fats.

- Protein is necessary for the development of lean muscle tissue and ridding the body of fat.

- You don't have to be perfect. I know that there will be times that you don't eat five small meals each day. I just ask that you follow this system as closely as possible. As I mentioned in the beginning of this book, the more effort you put into this system, the more you will get out of it.

Chapter V

Cheating is legal!

Chuck, the cheater

C huck was in his early fifties, and a large man. He had tried many different ways to lose weight and feel better including weight loss centers, fad diets and health clubs, but none of these methods worked for him. Chuck felt hopeless. He told me, "I need a solution that will work for good. No more quick fixes!"

Chuck was following my system well and didn't have any problem eating frequently or eating foods in the correct proportions. I was proud of him. I also discovered that he was an animal in the gym! He wasn't as strong as he had been in his twenties and thirties, but he worked out with more intensity than the next two people combined. He really wanted to improve his health and fitness.

Chuck was initially hesitant when I told him to use a "cheat day." He felt he should eat well all the time, and believed a cheat day would sabotage his results. I told him how important it was both mentally and physically to spend one day a week, eating whatever you desire in moderation. It's a great way to "reset" your system.

Chuck started using the cheat day and began to enjoy the concept. He would eat well all week long and then reward himself on Sunday with wherever he desired. He told me, "This isn't a bad system after all!"

Chuck began to see and feel results. He lost inches around his waist, his clothes fit better and he was able to move with less pain in his joints and muscles. He was thrilled!

However, Chuck began to stray from the system. He no longer used a cheat day. Instead, he spread out his cheat day over many days. He rationalized if he had a "cheat" lunch on Tuesday, a "cheat" dinner on Thursday and some "cheat" drinks during happy hour on Friday, it would be the same as combining them all on one day.

I became aware of this behavior during our monthly testing session. I regularly perform tests that include taking a percentage of body fat, girth measurements and lean body mass. Chuck's results had consistently been positive for two straight months. However, his results were negative this month. His body fat percentage and girth measurements had increased.

Chuck had still been attacking his workouts with intensity, so I knew that he didn't need a kick in the butt to increase his motivation. Upon examining Chuck's nutrition in detail, I recognized the cheating problem. He explained his rationale. He was having three to four cheat days a week and his body was suffering the consequences. It was time to explain to Chuck why this behavior was detrimental.

I told Chuck that his current eating behavior was "trapping" fat on his body. He was still working out hard, but his nutrition was not supporting the development of his lean muscle tissue. The frequency of his cheating was prohibiting his body from consistently utilizing his fat for energy. He was consuming too much simple sugar and spiking his insulin too frequently to lose fat.

Chuck appreciatived this new information. In fact, he made me a promise. He said, "Now that I know what I did wrong, I PROMISE I will consistently drop fat every month."

Since the time Chuck modified his cheat days and made his promise, he dropped his waistline a massive five inches in just four months! Also, he lowered his body fat by 5.5 percent and increased his lean body mass by eleven pounds. His jacket went from size fifty-four to forty-six. Chuck was ecstatic. He learned how to use his cheat day properly and reaped the rewards.

Cheating is legal!

Clients have often asked me, "Can I ever eat the desserts and rich foods that I love?" Absolutely! I believe that it is very important to eat whatever you enjoy or crave. If you deprive yourself of any type of food altogether, you will binge sooner or later and compromise your efforts. I recommend that you take one day a week and make it your cheat day. Just *one* day!

On your cheat day, eat whatever you desire, in moderation. For example, eat a piece or two of pizza, but not the whole pie. Eat a piece of cake, but not the whole sheet. It is still *very important* to eat frequently on your cheat day. You don't want to slow down your metabolism.

I've had some clients who initially say, "I don't need a cheat day; I'll be perfect all the time." I strongly warn you against not taking your cheat day. Sooner or later (we're all human) you will break down and binge.

I've seen clients go more than two months of eating perfectly, and then all hell breaks loose. They have deprived themselves so much they can rationalize eating anything. They get off their "game plan" and sometimes never recover.

Please use your cheat day to let off some steam and pressure. When you eat poorly after you have consistently eaten supportively, you'll feel awful and look forward to the next day when you can eat supportively again. So, again, I encourage you, use your cheat day.

It's important to eat whatever you like one day a week.

If you want to continue to burn fat quickly and efficiently, limit your cheat day to one specific day each week. For example, make every Saturday or Sunday your cheat day. I recommend that you use one day on the weekend as a cheat day because it is usually easier to eat more supportively during the week when you are on a schedule.

Cheating is legal!

Summary

- Incorporate one "cheat day" into your supportive eating habits.

- On your cheat day, eat whatever you want, in moderation.

- Meal frequency is important even on your cheat day.

Chapter VI

All fat is not created equally!

Faye, the fat eliminator

Faye was one of the most genuinely nice clients I've ever had the privilege of working with. She worked hard at everything she did in the gym because athletics didn't come naturally to her. Faye, like many clients, was primarily interested in losing body fat and shaping her body.

When I work with new clients I typically begin their first two to three weeks by focusing on weight training, a moderate amount of cardiovascular training and eating small frequent meals. This initiates their development of lean muscle tissue and speeds their metabolism. Faye worked very hard and was progressing nicely in this introductory phase.

The next phase of my system introduces more detailed nutritional education. Faye understood the importance of eating small frequent meals. She knew this would speed up her metabolism, and also knew the significance of combining a lean protein source, a slow-releasing carbohydrate and a green vegetable into each meal. The only question that Faye had was, "How many grams of fat should I eat a day?"

I answered Faye by asking a question: "What kind of fats are you referring to—saturated, unsaturated or essential fatty acids?"

She didn't know the difference between them and, like many, had read in the news that fat is bad. In fact, it has been promoted, mostly by food manufacturers, that fat must be eliminated altogether in order to lose weight and live "healthier." Unfortunately, nothing could be further from the truth.

I explained to Faye that all fat is not the same. Obviously, the fat found in doughnuts isn't the same and isn't as beneficial to you as fat found in freshwater fish like salmon or swordfish. *All* fat is high in calories and contain nine calories per gram. Remember, protein and carbohydrates contain just four calories per gram. However, the body uses saturated and unsaturated fat differently. The body doesn't have much use for saturated fat. It's the "bad" fat that clogs arteries. On the other hand, the body does have a need for unsaturated and, more specifically, polyunsaturated essential fat. These omega fats include flax oil, fish oil, hemp oil and safflower oil. This is "good" fat that is necessary to help you achieve your health and fitness goals.

The reason these fats are called essential fatty acids is because

Flax oil is a great source of essential fatty acids.

the body doesn't make them naturally. If the body doesn't get these fats from foods, lean muscle tissue will be broken down to get them. As you know, lean muscle tissue is important. If lean muscle tissue is broken down, your metabolism will work slower. This would be detrimental to your results, as it was to Faye's.

I recommended that Faye avoid saturated fat and hydrogenated oils such as butter, peanut butter, margarine and vegetable oil. I also suggested she take a serving of flax oil or ground flax seeds daily. These essential fatty acids help protect lean muscle tissue, control sugar cravings and regulate insulin.

Faye discovered how various fats react differently within the body. She also learned the importance of essential fatty acids and how they help protect lean muscle tissue. After she incorporated good fat into her nutritional program, she proceeded to drop her body fat by thirteen percent in ten months. She also gained more muscle tone and increased her energy level to the point where she felt like a kid again!

Avoid saturated fats and hydrogenated oils.

All fat is not created equally!

Americans have heard for the past fifteen years that they should limit fat intake, especially saturated fats. Notice that I said *limit* intake, not eliminate fat altogether. This is because fat is an *essential* macronutrient. The word essential means that dietary fat is necessary for basic processes of the body to occur and the body cannot produce these fats by itself.

I strongly recommend that my clients consume flax, fish or hemp oil daily. These essential fatty acids (EFAs) contain omega oils which help stabilize blood sugar and provide a satisfied or satiated feeling to the mind and body. This will facilitate the reduction of sugar cravings and help complete the amino acid (protein building block) chains necessary for the regeneration of lean muscle tissue.

It is important to limit *saturated* fats (fats that are solid at room temperature) like butter and lard, as well as fatty cuts of meat. It is also important to stay away from "hydrogenated" oils such as those contained in most peanut butters and margarines. These foods don't contain essential fatty acids. The body can easily make saturated fats from carbohydrates. Therefore, it isn't necessary to consume saturated fats. You should avoid them whenever possible, for they aren't supportive of a lean, toned and healthy body.

Remember, even though some fats are essential, fats are still high in calories. For example, one gram of fat equals nine calories, while one gram of carbohydrates and protein has just four calories. Also, as discussed earlier, fats have a low thermal effect. The calories of fat that you consume are not utilized as efficiently as proteins and complex carbohydrates in the breakdown of food.

Calories per gram of specific macronutrients

Proteins	4
Carbohydrates	4
Fats	9

Summary

- The body requires essential fatty acids (EFAs) such as flax, fish and hemp oils, *not* saturated fats and hydrogenated oils.

- One gram of fat contains nine calories.

- One gram of protein or carbohydrates contains just four calories.

Chapter VII

Sugar warning!

Monica, the sugarholic

Monica was in her late fifties and new to exercise. Her primary goal was to lose "a lot" of weight, as she was about five feet nine inches and 260 pounds. She told me that she had been active most of her life enjoying golf, tennis and skiing, but when she hit forty-five years old, her metabolism and her activity level, just seemed to stop. She told me nutrition was not a problem because she ate "right." She then said she would follow any type of exercise training I recommend.

I've learned to question everything. If someone tells me they have been active and exercising I want to know what kind of exercise and how often. If someone says they eat "right," I want to know how they define eating right. I asked Monica to describe to me her typical day of nutrition.

She started off by telling me she eats a raisin and bran cereal with a banana and orange juice for breakfast every morning. She sometimes has an apple for a snack between breakfast and lunch. For lunch she usually has a sandwich with low fat turkey or ham and fat free cheese on a roll. For dinner she eats pasta or chicken and rice or some type of meat and potato. I asked her if she snacks after dinner and she said, "Sometimes, but always low fat products like cookies or pretzels."

Before I criticize or comment on someone's nutrition, I always ask, "How important is it for you to lose fat and regain your health?" Monica said, "It's very important." I asked, "Are you willing to do what it takes to accomplish your goals?" She replied, "Yes, whatever it takes." I said, "The primary reason you have gained so much body fat and weight over the last few years is for two reasons. First, as the body ages it loses muscle tissue and, consequently, your metabolism slows down. Secondly, you are eating about eighty to ninety percent of your calories from sugar."

Monica thought and then said, "I never eat candy or drink soda pop. How can I be eating too much sugar?" I proceeded to describe the three primary macronutrients: protein, carbohydrates and fats. I emphasized to Monica that *all* carbohydrates are sugar. However, the body uses simple carbohydrates and complex carbohydrates differently. Simple carbohydrates like juice, candy, fruit and soda pop immediately spike blood sugar levels and cause an insulin response. Also, most enriched carbohydrates like white rice, white pasta and white bread also spike blood sugar levels because they are enriched with sugar.

I explained to Monica that the cereal, fruit, bread, pasta, juice, pretzels and low fat cookies are all *loaded* with simple enriched sugar. I didn't tell her to eliminate these foods forever. I just wanted her to understand that these foods won't help to lower body fat, lose scale weight or even increase long-term energy.

Complex carbohydrates and, more specifically, slow-releasing complex carbohydrates that contain no enriched sugar don't spike blood sugar levels as much or quickly. Therefore, slow-releasing complex carbohydrates don't cause as much of an insulin response. This helps the body sustain long-term energy and utilize fat more efficiently.

I recommended to Monica that she begin to replace simple carbohydrates and enriched white carbohydrates with slow-releasing carbohydrates like wheat pasta, brown rice and wheat bread. Next, I recommended the reduction of all carbohydrates, including slow-releasing ones, to approximately forty percent of her caloric intake. This percentage may vary per individual dependant upon goals, physical condition and age.

Lean protein sources and green vegetables should replace the excess amount of carbohydrates in her daily eating habits. I reiterated the importance of eating a lean protein source, a slow-releasing carbohydrate and a vegetable every three to three and a half hours.

Finally, I insisted that Monica must continue to weight train and perform a moderate amount of cardiovascular training three times a week. Remember, lean muscle tissue is the only place in the body where fat and calories are burned. Since Monica is post-menopausal and has lost considerable lean muscle tissue, weight training is essential for the achievement of her goals.

Monica is continuing to work hard to meet her goals, and is still a work in progress. She currently has reduced her body fat five percent in four months and has lost twenty pounds of scale weight. She knows she has a long way to go and is committed to attaining results. I continuously encourage Monica to work hard, eat well and be patient. She's doing better every day.

Sugar warning!

Simple carbohydrates (sugar) are a different concern from fat altogether. The consumption of sugar is necessary for energy. However, I've seen hundreds of clients dramatically transform their bodies by avoiding most simple and some complex sugar. I've read agricultural reports that indicate the average American consumes between 150 to 180 pounds of sugar per year! And that's what the *average* American consumes. Just think how much sugar those who are not aware or careful of their nutrition consume in a year!

Limit your sugar consumption.

Whenever you consume sugar, whether simple or complex, your blood sugar level will increase. Provided that you aren't diabetic, your body will produce a hormone called insulin to regulate this increase in blood sugar level. Your body needs to keep its blood sugar level within a normal range of 90 to 120 mg/dl.

When your body releases insulin in response to blood sugar ingestion, it often over-regulates the blood sugar, driving it below the normal range. This low sugar level then causes a sugar craving. Consequently, you may feel the need to eat additional sources of sugar to satisfy this internal condition.

This additional sugar will again spike blood sugar and cause the release of more insulin. So you will crave even more sugar! This cycle explains the "sweet tooth" you may experience after dinner. A "sweet tooth" isn't genetic, and isn't something that is only germane to you or your family. It's the craving of sugar due to the insulin response, an addictive cycle from which most people cannot break free. This is exactly why many Americans accumulate fat and become obese.

Glucagon is another important hormone; however, it works in an inverse relationship to insulin. When the body produces insulin, it can't produce glucagon. The detrimental aspect here is that glucagon is one of the hormones that helps burn and oxidize fat. Therefore, whenever you eat sugar your body goes through the insulin response cycle. The body is then prevented from producing glucagon and burning fat. Thus, *you cannot burn fat when you are consuming most sugars.* You're trapping fat in your body!

Some slow-releasing complex carbohydrates, such as brown rice and sweet potatoes, do not cause *as quick* a change in the blood sugar level compared to simple fast-releasing carbohydrates. Thus the body does not need as much insulin as quickly to regulate the blood sugar level. Most fast sugar releasing complex carbohydrates cause a dramatic spike in blood sugar and more insulin is required to regulate it. These foods include most enriched white complex carbohydrates such as white bread, bagels, dough, white pasta, white rice, pretzels, white crackers and white potatoes. Fast sugar releasing complex carbohydrates cause a similar response in your blood sugar as simple carbohydrates (sugar) such as table sugar, fruit, candy and honey.

Fast-releasing complex carbohydrates are not supportive of stabilizing blood sugar levels and reducing your body fat. However, whether fast- or slow-releasing,

Though vegetables contain carbohydrates, most don't dramatically elevate blood sugar levels. Vegetables are essential and should be consumed at least twice daily.

it is important not to consume too much of any kind of carbohydrate. This is because a large quantity of any carbohydrate will cause an insulin response.

A growing health problem in this country is type two diabetes, also known as adult onset diabetes. The development of this condition is due in part to poor nutritional habits, inadequate exercise and increasing body fat. The American Diabetes Association, in its 1999 Annual Report, states that type two diabetes is "a metabolic disorder resulting from the body's inability to make enough, or properly use, insulin. It is the most common form of the disease. Type two diabetes accounts for ninety to ninety-five percent of diabetes. Type two diabetes is nearing epidemic proportions, due to an increased number of older Americans and a greater prevalence of obesity and sedentary lifestyles." Through the reduction of body fat, eating supportive meals frequently, and developing lean muscle tissue, you may greatly decrease your chances of developing type two diabetes.

If a product doesn't say "sugar" in the ingredients list, it doesn't mean that it's sugar-free. Sugar comes in many forms. If you read food labels, be on the lookout for the ingredients listed below.

Various Types of Simple Sugars

Glucose	Fructose
Corn syrup	Barley malt
Glycerin	Maltose
Honey	Sucrose
Fruit extracts	Dextrin
Cellulose	Lactose
Levulose	Aorbitol
Xylitol	Mannitol

The items listed above are all examples of simple sugars. Marketers love to hide these sugars in the ingredients list. However, if you read the ingredients list and know some of their tricks, you'll be less apt to be fooled by these sneaky devils.

Many Americans have a growing concern about using artificial sweeteners. When artificial sweeteners are substituted for sugar, your body will be able to reduce its body fat more efficiently and forego the insulin response cycle. Over time, this may reduce your chance of developing obesity and/or type two diabetes. As far as the safety of using artificial sweeteners, I believe they are safe when used in moderation. In their 1999 Annual Report, the American Diabetes Association approved the use of three artificial sweeteners in moderate amounts: saccharin, aspartame and acesulfame potassium. I tell my clients to use diet drinks and artificial sweeteners instead of sugar-based drinks or sugar, but to do so in moderation.

Break yourself free from sugar!

If you are a bit of a sugarholic—and most of us are from time to time—you need to do something that is going to be difficult. You need to give up sugar for three days, eat the way I recommend and exercise. If you do these things, I PROMISE that your sugar cravings will diminish. The first day will be somewhat uncomfortable, since your body is conditioned to having excess sugar in its system.

The second day will be even more challenging and you could even get a headache, and the third day will be the most difficult. You may want to break down and give into the craving, but hold fast. The end is near! By the fourth day you will no longer crave sugars. You will have broken free from the physical addiction.

Now, I'm not saying that you'll never desire chocolate chip cookies or ice cream again. I don't believe that you should ever give up anything you enjoy forever. However, you'll notice a change in your tastes and appetite. You'll begin to desire foods such as brown rice and green vegetables (hard to believe, but true!), and you'll soon enjoy good lean sources of protein. Believe it or

Because of the effect alcohol has on blood sugar, it is important to limit your consumption to two drinks per week.

not, you'll learn to listen to your body and nourish it with foods that will support your goals.

Alcohol

My clients often want to know what effect alcohol has on gaining or losing body fat. Alcohol, whether it's beer, wine or hard liquor, is comprised of alcohol and sugar. Both of these ingredients will significantly affect your blood sugar and insulin, and thus your body fat.

In the *Quebec Family Study*, alcohol intake was associated with a high daily caloric intake and fat gain, particularly in the trunk area. Tremblay and Cigolini, in their paper, "Body fatness in active individuals reporting low lipid and alcohol intake," reported the finding of "a positive association between usual alcohol ingestion and body fat accumulation at the trunk." I usually tell my clients they are free to consume up to two servings of alcohol a week. Any more than that will make the reduction of body fat difficult.

Fruit

A concept many of my clients have a hard time understanding is the adverse consequences of consuming fruit. You've been told for most of your life that any type of fruit is good to eat at any time. Also, you've heard if you eat a lot of fruit and lay off junk food, you

Remember, fruit is sugar and consumption yields an insulin response.

will lose weight. I want you to be aware that fruit is sugar! Fructose, or fruit sugar, reacts in the body with insulin and glucagon just like sucrose, honey, or table sugar, so your body can't differentiate between the sugar in an apple and the sugar in a Snickers bar! I'm not saying that you can never eat fruit. What I am saying is that you should know that the consumption of fruit will affect your blood sugar levels and insulin secretion. Sugar from fruit is as addictive as sugar from candy or white bread, and the consumption of it makes it very difficult to lower your body fat. I typically reserve eating fruit for my cheat day. So if your goal is to lose fat and inches, eat fruit sparingly.

Sugar warning!

Summary

- Sugar causes an insulin response that ultimately leads to fat gain.

- Always check the ingredients list of foods so that you are less likely to be deceived by slick marketers.

- Consume no more than two servings of alcohol per week.

- Fruit is a simple sugar, so limit your consumption.

Chapter VIII

Don't be fooled by slick marketers

Daryl, the duped

Daryl came to me as a last hope. He had tried all of the weight loss programs before; in fact, he told me that his attempts included weight loss centers, low protein diets, low fat diets, cabbage soup diets, frivolous home fitness equipment, aerobic classes, health club memberships, over-the-counter metabolism-increasing pills, and prescription fat blockers. He also attempted to eat "fat free," "low fat" and "reduced fat." He only bought foods that were "natural," "lean" and "light."

After listening to Daryl share for half an hour what he had tried to lose weight and shape and tone his body, I was dizzy! Simultaneously, I felt sympathy for him. It wasn't his fault he was out of shape. He tried very hard to take control of his body and health, but by listening to bad advice. Unfortunately, he'll *never* get into shape following this ineffective information. He, as well as millions of other individuals, had been misinformed and deceived by marketers. Misinformation and deception in the health and fitness industry is the main reason why I developed this system and wrote this book.

After listening to Daryl's sad but common story, I began to educate him on why his attempts hadn't been successful. I said, "Daryl, you didn't fail. You've been deceived into trying what you wanted to believe!" Products are manufactured and marketed to sell and make money. Consequently, there is widespread deception in this industry.

I informed Daryl that he would only need three things to get into the best shape and health of his life: weight training, eating supportive meals frequently and performing cardiovascular training in moderation. I told him to forget about everything else he thought he knew about losing fat and scale weight. I said, "Unlike what marketers boast, it isn't quick, it isn't easy and it doesn't work 'like magic'! There's no special exercise machine that burns fat quicker, and there are no magic metabolism increasing pills. Diets don't work long-term and food manufacturers want to sell their fat free and low fat products."

Daryl stopped me and said, "I understand how I've been deceived with exercise machines and magic pills, but I'm not sure that food manufacturers can legally mislead the public with regards to their products." Daryl's comment was good. How can food manufacturers legally deceive and misinform the public?

I explained to him that food manufacturers want their products to sell. Since most people want to eat well, a product that claims to be fat free sounds more appealing than a product that doesn't. Food manufacturers know this and use loopholes in the labeling laws to market their products. The most common loophole has to do with serving sizes. For example, a product can be labeled fat free if it has less than .5 grams of fat per serving. Food manufacturers can get any product to be less than .5 grams per serving if they make the serving size small enough. Check the serving size of fat free cooking oil or low fat cookies. You may be surprised!

I also warned Daryl that, just because a product is labeled fat free, it doesn't mean it's supportive of your goals to lose fat and scale weight. It's important to know that dietary fat and body fat are two separate things. You can gain or lose body fat independently of eating fat free, low fat or reduced fat. In fact, most fat free products contain very high portions of sugar to give them a better taste. Fat free cookies are an excellent example of high concentrations of sugar added to replace fat in the product.

I instructed Daryl to disregard food label hype. I told him to read the ingredients list on the back of the package and discover what is truly in the product. If a product is high in sugar, it won't be supportive of your goals. If a product has a tiny serving size, it's important not to overuse the product because it will be high in calories. Always read the ingredients and serving size. They'll reveal the contents of the product.

Don't be fooled by slick marketers

Food manufacturers know one thing: how to make money by selling food. The words they put on their labels entice you to purchase their product, for example, "Light," "Low Fat," "Fat Free," "Reduced Fat," "Lean" and "Healthy." However, these foods might not resemble anything close to what I categorized earlier as supportive. Don't let the slick product marketers fool you into believing you are purchasing a product that will help you improve your health and fitness. I'll teach you some tips to help avoid being seduced by these tricky manufacturers.

First, when you shop for food, I suggest that you limit your purchases to the perimeter of the store. This is where you will find staple items such as meat, fish, eggs, poultry and vegetables. This suggestion alone will save you hundreds of dollars each year on deceitful, misleading and wrongly labeled garbage. You will not only save money, you'll also save time and extra inches on your waistline.

Next, it's important to have a grocery list already prepared before you start shopping (see Chapter XVI). If a food isn't on the list, don't buy it. If a food wasn't important or supportive to you when you prepared the list, it still isn't important or supportive when you see the bright colorful packaging and deceptive label. Don't buy it!

How do food manufacturers get away with their deceptive claims? Let's take a closer look.

"Fat Free"

Many food labels have the words "fat free" plastered all over their packaging—for one reason only. Those words *sell products*. In fact, I read a report in the *New England Journal of Medicine* that states that each year, food manufacturers produce over 50,000 new products claiming to be fat free, low fat, reduced fat or light. Does the label accurately represent what ingredients are in the product? In far too many cases, absolutely not. The label has little to do with the ingredients or quality of the food being sold, but it has everything to do with the bottom line and increased profits. Do you really think that food manufacturers are looking out for your best interest or theirs?

Hundreds of new low fat products are introduced into stores each years.

You'll find out if you go to the grocery store, or perhaps only as far as your refrigerator, and look at one of the "fat free" butter substitutes. Look at the ingredients. You will likely find the main ingredient is hydrogenated oil. Hydrogenated oils are pure fat! So how do the labelers get away with calling a product that is pure fat, fat free? Labeling laws have been created with massive loopholes that allow food manufacturers to mislead or, in some cases, blatantly lie about their products. The loophole usually involves the serving size. If a product has less than .5 grams of fat *per serving*, the product can legally be labeled fat free. How do you think that food manufacturers can get any product to have less than .5 grams of fat per serving? The answer is by decreasing the serving size under .5 grams! The law doesn't define how small a serving size can be. Consequently, manufacturers can label all their products fat free if their serving size is small enough.

This is seen most clearly in sprayed cooking oil. Cooking oil, or any oil for that matter, is by definition 100 percent fat. However, many manufacturers of cooking oil label their products as fat free. If you look at the serving size, you will discover that the suggested serving size is a one-third-second spray! I've tried many times, and maybe you're better than me, but I can't hold the nozzle one-third of a second. I either get nothing out or the spray lasts at least one second. If the spray is one second, I'm consuming three serving sizes according to the manufacturer. Some clients tell me they hold their spray long enough to coat the pan. In my estimation, that's at least three seconds. Three seconds of spray is nine servings! Also, the manufacturer claims that there are 550 servings per container. I defy anyone to get 550 equal servings out of that aerosol container.

"95 Percent Fat Free"

This has always been one of my favorites. If you were to eat a stick of butter (please don't do it!), you would be consuming 100 percent of your calories from fat. If you were to take the same stick of butter and mix it with water and then drink the solution, you would still be getting 100 percent of your calories from fat, since water doesn't contain any calories.

If you were a food manufacturer and you wanted to sell your butter/water solution to health-conscious consumers, you wouldn't sell much if you put the words "100 percent of calories from fat" on the label. However, you could be a little tricky and modify the solution to have the same amount of butter and water by *volume*, not by calories. You could then label your product as fifty percent fat

Look at the serving size of products.

Manufacturers add water to reduce the fat in milk.

free by volume. Even though 100 percent of the calories is still from fat, the law doesn't stipulate that you cannot label by volume. If fifty percent fat free doesn't sound good enough, no problem! More water can be added to get whatever percentage you desire, such as ninety-five percent fat free. Now that sounds more appealing, doesn't it?

And don't think that only butter is manipulated. Meats and poultry are also commonly pumped with water to reduce the fat by volume on the label. However, the biggest target for years has been milk. Milk is mostly water and 100 percent of the calories come from fat. You commonly see milk labeled as skim (no fat), one percent fat, two percent fat or whole (which they claim is five percent fat). The only difference in any milk product is the amount of water that is added. Skim milk has the most water added, thus, it is nearly fat free by volume. However, don't be deceived. No type of milk has less than forty percent of its calories from fat! It's deceptive, but it sells.

Before you get all worked up about the fact the food industry has been lying to you for years—and, by the way, let me tell you it has—you can't possibly fight against them. There's too much money involved. Senators and congressmen are given billions of dollars each year by political action coalitions and lobbyists, such as food manufacturers, to ensure the laws don't change.

I suggest you educate yourself instead of fighting the food industry. You can't save the nation, but you can educate yourself and your family. It is crucial to know how food manufacturers manipulate product labels. Don't let yourself be deceived by their slick marketing strategies. This knowledge will help you immensely in improving your health and fitness.

So how do you see through the deceptive labeling?

On any food label, manufacturers are required to list ingredients in *descending order of abundance*. If any item in that list includes fat (oil, lard, butter, whole milk, etc.), you can't be looking at a fat free product, regardless of what the marketers claim in big print on the package.

Manufacturers are also required to list the number of calories per serving and the number of calories from fat, protein and carbohydrates. First, find the serving size on the label and make sure it's more than .5 grams. Then *ignore* the section providing percentage of daily value because it refers to what the government believes the percentage breakdown would be of proteins, carbohydrates and fats based on a 2,000 calorie a day diet. Who said anything about 2,000 calories a day? And how does the government know what our nutritional goals are?

Divide the number of calories from fat by the total number of calories per serving to determine what percentage of the food is fat. For example, if a label indicates that the food contains 100 calories per serving, and thirty calories are from fat, it is easy to see that the food is thirty percent fat. The same calculations can be done for carbohydrates and protein.

You can also use the grams per serving to determine the percentage of calories contained in a product. You've already learned that each gram of fat contains nine calories and protein and carbohydrates contain four calories per gram. So,

Nutrition Facts		
Serving size: 1/2 cup		
Servings per container: 2		
Amount Per Serving		
Calories 180	Calories from Fat 90	
		% Daily Value
Total fat 10g		15%
Saturated Fat 4g		20%
Cholesterol 0mg		0%
Sodium 0mg		0%
Total Carbohydrates 10.5g		4%
Sugars 2g		
Protein 12g		

Summary of percentage of fat by calories

- Product contains 10g of fat per serving and 180 calories per serving.

- Each gram of fat contains nine calories.

- Calories of fat per serving = 10 x 9 = 90.

- Percentage of fat per serving is 180/90 = .5 or 50 percent.

if a product has ten grams of fat per serving, multiply ten by nine and you will get ninety. That equals ninety calories of fat per serving. If the total number of calories per serving were 180, then ninety divided by 180 would be .5 or fifty percent fat.

I would suggest for any product that it is important to keep overall fat intake down to twenty-five to thirty percent per serving unless the product is an essential fatty acid. If a product is more than thirty percent fat by serving, it can be harmful to the body and to your fitness results because of the high caloric density.

"Sugar Free"

By now I hope you're becoming much less trusting of labels. Good! By knowing the tricks of food manufacturers and how the labeling laws work or better yet, don't work, you're leaning how to protect yourself. As many of my clients know, the gross over- consumption of sugar is one of the biggest reasons why people get fat.

Being from Buffalo, New York—birthplace of the Buffalo chicken wing and home to *long* winters—I see "fatness" or, to use the medical term, "adiposity" every day. I see obese, overweight and out-of-shape people everywhere. They're typically drinking a soda (not a diet soda!), orange juice or, better yet, a beer! They may be eating bagels, pretzels, pizza, popcorn or some other type of enriched starchy white carbohydrate. Let me re-emphasize—if you consume more than a moderate amount of sugar, you will gain body fat. I PROMISE!

Watch out for products that contain large amounts of sugar.

To give you some specific examples, a twenty-ounce bottle of Coke contains 100 calories per serving and two and a half servings per container. So if you drink the entire container (which isn't that hard to do), you'll consume 250 calories. Coke contains twenty-seven grams of sugar per serving. Now remember, there are two and a half servings per container, so that equals 67.5 grams of sugar for a twenty-ounce bottle of Coke.

Maybe you didn't know this, but one teaspoon of sugar is equivalent to four grams. So if you divide 67.5 grams by four teaspoons per gram, the twenty-ounce bottle of Coke contains almost seventeen teaspoons of sugar! Most of us would never dream of sitting in front of the sugar bowl and eating seventeen straight teaspoons of sugar. It would be awful! Sickening! However, many of us would not hesitate to consume one if not more Coca-Colas per day. It's no wonder, then, sixty-one percent of Americans were defined as overweight according to a report published by the Centers for Disease Control in January 2001.

You might be thinking to yourself, "Well, that's soda pop. I never drink soda." If you don't drink soda, good. Soda won't do anything to support your muscle and it will create havoc with your insulin response. You will also gain body fat. However, soda pop is not the only product that contains a deceptive amount of sugar.

Let's take a look at orange juice. A common brand of orange juice contains 120 calories per serving and two servings per sixteen-ounce bottle. Therefore, the entire sixteen ounces of juice contains 240 calories. Also, this bottle of orange juice contains thirty-one grams of sugar per serving or sixty-one grams total. Once again, if you divide sixty-one grams of sugar by four teaspoons per gram, you get 15.25 teaspoons in the bottle of juice! Since the juice has 15.25 teaspoons of sugar per sixteen-ounce bottle and Coke has seventeen teaspoons per twenty-ounce bottle, the juice contains *more sugar per ounce* than Coke! As I mentioned before, if you want to lose fat, you must carefully examine the labels of products you consume.

	Coke	Orange Juice
Size in ounces	20	16
Calories	250	240
Grams of sugar	67.5	61
Teaspoons of sugar	17	15.25
Teaspoons of sugar per ounce	.85	.95

A sixteen-ounce orange juice contains more than fifteen teaspoons of sugar!

I've seen packages with labels that indicate that the enclosed brownies are "sugar free," yet the most prominent ingredient is fructose. Sure, it's fruit sugar and marketers can call it natural; however, it's still sugar. Remember that simple sugars include glucose, fructose, corn syrup, barley malt, glycerin, glycerol, honey, sucrose, and fruit extracts. It's in your best interest to avoid (or at least limit) consumption.

Don't be fooled by slick marketers

Summary

- Look at product labels to see if manufacturers are "sneaking" fats and sugars into the ingredients list.

- Remember, food manufacturers' intention is to persuade you to purchase their product, sometimes with less than honest claims.

- Consuming too much sugar or fat will increase your body fat and jeopardize your health and fitness goals.

Chapter IX

Aerobic exercise can make you fatter

Mary, the aerobic freak

Mary arranged a consultation with me about losing weight and toning her body. She was somewhat different than many people with whom I typically consult. She wasn't a novice exerciser and had attended various health clubs for years. She knew the importance of exercise for both her health and fitness. I said to Mary, "I understand that you've been exercising for years. In what ways would you like me to help you?" As she grabbed her butt, Mary responded, "I want to know exactly what I have to do to tone my body and lose *this*!"

I asked her what she had been doing. She told me that she had been doing one hour of cardiovascular training every Monday, Wednesday, and Friday on either the treadmill or the stair stepper. On Tuesdays, Thursdays and Saturdays she attended step aerobic classes that lasted about ninety minutes. Before I could respond, she blurted out, "Do you think that I should increase my cardio time on Mondays, Wednesdays and Fridays, or should I do additional cardio on Sunday?"

I calmly asked her, "Do you want to get a fatter fanny?" Mary was shocked and said, "What do you mean?" I proceeded to explain to her that she was constantly breaking down her muscle tissue.

This woman was doing seven and a half hours of cardiovascular training a week! The huge amount of cardio was burning her muscle as energy. I explained to her that the less muscle tissue she has on her body, the fewer calories and fat she will burn. Further, I tried to impress upon her the fact she was actually *slowing down* her metabolism by doing so much cardiovascular training.

Many exercisers are similar to Mary and inaccurately believe that more exercise is better. If spending twenty-five minutes doing aerobic training is good, forty-five minutes must be better. Some misinformed people also think, "I want to get into the best shape as quickly as I can, so I'll do sixty minutes of aerobic training every day." I urge you not to fall victim to this misconception. I'll repeat again: it is *essential*, in order to speed your metabolism and lower your body fat, that you don't exercise away your muscle tissue by doing *too much* cardiovascular training!

Aerobic exercise can make you fatter

What if you're really committed to getting into better shape? Let's say that you're absolutely dedicated to dropping fat and "sweating off" the weight. You're faithfully walking forty minutes on the treadmill and performing aerobic step class four to five days a week.

You're really trying hard and are doing everything in your power to finally get in shape. How do you think you would you feel at the end of a month if you were actually fatter than before you started this difficult exercise program? I think that you'd feel cheated and angry. I believe that you might never go to the gym again. You might feel that exercise doesn't work and isn't right for you. In this

Maintain your lean muscle tissue by performing aerobic training in moderation.

chapter, I will explain how cardiovascular exercise can make you fatter and how my system will prevent you from ever having this happen.

Cardiovascular and aerobic exercises are the same and I will uses these terms interchangeably throughout this book. The question is, how can increased cardiovascular exercise make you fatter? Please stay with me while I try to simplify this as much as possible.

When you eat complex carbohydrates, they're slowly converted into glucose and stored in the muscle as glycogen, which is a fuel reserve for your muscles. Glycogen stores are limited, so if you don't eat sufficiently to keep those stores full, your aerobic session may exhaust your stored sugar. If this happens, your body will tap into muscle to create its own fuel by converting some amino acids (the building blocks of muscle and protein) into sugars that can provide the fuel needed for body functions.

The only way your body can access those amino acids is to break down muscle tissue. Thus it is possible during aerobic exercise to exercise away precious muscle tissue. By now, you understand that this will have a long-term negative effect, making your body more efficient at storing fat!

I am *not* suggesting that you don't perform aerobic exercise. In fact, in The Promise Fat Loss & Fitness System, I recommend you include aerobic exercise several times per week. However, it's vital to perform aerobic exercise in moderation. The specific amount of time you spend doing aerobic exercise actually depends upon your physical condition, the amount of muscle that you have and your fitness goals.

For example, if you've been lifting weights, have good muscle tone and low body fat, you should probably never exceed fifteen to twenty minutes of aerobic activity at one time in order to preserve your lean muscle tissue. On the other hand, if you're relatively new to weight training, have limited muscle tone and body fat above eighteen percent for men and twenty percent for women, you could probably perform up to thirty to thirty-five minutes of aerobic exercise per session without breaking down a significant amount of your lean muscle tissue.

The exact amount of desirable aerobic training varies on an individual basis according to the factors mentioned above. If you aren't sure whether you're performing too much or too little aerobic training, contact a personal fitness professional for assistance.

For those of you who belong to a health club or have ever been in a health club before, I want you to visualize people exercising. You can probably recollect that the majority of the people exercising were performing cardiovascular exercise. The stair steppers were full, the elliptical climbers were humming and there was probably even a line and sign-up sheet to use the treadmills. If you can picture the people using this equipment, were most of them lean and toned or soft and flabby? I've found most of them to have higher amounts of body fat and many were significantly out-of-shape or obese.

Now I want you to visualize the people who were using the free weights. Probably less than ten percent of the people in the gym were in this area rather than in the aerobic area. Younger men, some women and a few determined individuals working with a personal trainer mostly inhabit this area. Were most of the people in the free weight area lean and toned or soft and flabby? I've found, and I'm sure you'll agree, the majority of them are lean and toned. They have developed lean muscle tissue and generally appear to be in good shape.

Do you want to work out like people who are soft and flabby or lean and toned? I know you want "less jiggle and more ripple." So work out with free weights and perform a limited amount of cardiovascular training.

Anytime you perform aerobic activities, your body has three options for fuel. It can burn blood sugar, fat or muscle. If your blood sugar is fluctuating due to going long periods without supportive nutrition, your body will release less fat. If you consume simple sugars, fat release will be compromised due to insulin production. And if you don't take in enough calories to support your activity, your body will actually "cling" to fat and will cause aerobic movement to seek out sugar as a fuel source. Thus aerobic exercise may *not* utilize your stored body fat at all. *It may make you fatter!*

In Part III: Body in Motion, which includes the workout sections, you will clearly see the relationship between your time spent with weight training and cardiovascular training. On three days per week, I provide you with exact weight training exercises that will take you approximately thirty minutes to perform. I also provide you with precise information regarding a moderate amount of cardiovascular training six days a week. Don't worry. These workouts are within your capabilities and will maintain your interest. Remember, you now have the information and desire to succeed.

Aerobic exercise can make you fatter

Summary

- Perform cardiovascular training in moderation.

- Performing too much cardiovascular training may break down your muscle tissue. This will slow down your metabolism and make you fatter.

- Spend less time doing cardiovascular training and more time engaging in weight training.

- Contact a personal fitness professional if you have questions regarding weight training or cardiovascular training workouts.

Chapter X

Spend less time in the gym

Mary, the aerobic freak, part two

Returning to the discussion in the last chapter about Mary, I recommended that she perform cardiovascular training no more than three times per week for thirty minutes at a time. I also told her that she needed to do weight training three times a week and eat in a supportive manner. Mary's biggest concern was the concept of spending less time on the treadmill while attaining better results. She didn't believe it was possible to look better and lose more fat doing one and a half hours of cardiovascular training instead of seven and a half hours a week.

As you can imagine, this conversation was not as straightforward as I just described. The consultation took nearly ninety minutes. At the end of the consultation, she was still not completely convinced my recommendations would work.

I don't blame her. She was previously led to believe that the more cardiovascular training she performed, the more calories and fat she would burn. Mary was watching the calorie counter on the treadmill and equating it to the number of calories she believed she consumed in a day. By the way, the calorie counter on cardiovascular machines is just a gauge, something that equipment manufacturers have included on the machinery as a feature to occupy you.

Drop body fat and lose inches by doing aerobic training in moderation and spending less time in the gym.

It doesn't accurately measure your caloric output, so don't be concerned with it.

I finally convinced Mary to try The Promise Fat Loss & Fitness System for a few months. I PROMISED her that after two months of training with weights, doing less cardiovascular training and eating supportive meals frequently, she would dramatically reduce her body fat. In fact, I bet my reputation on it.

In just two months of training with me, she reduced her body fat 4.5 percent and dropped two inches around her waist and hips! Incidentally, she lost eleven pounds of scale weight, but I want to re-emphasize that scale weight means nothing. Mary had lost scale weight dozens of times before, but she never lowered her body fat and increased her metabolism. The reduction of scale weight is a byproduct of low body fat, but remember, it isn't the most critical issue. More importantly, she told me that, finally, her "a-- looked great in jeans!" She was thrilled. She found out how she could spend less time in the gym and get better results.

Spend less time in the gym

You're a busy person. I'm sure you have many career and personal commitments that keep you busy every day. You most likely can't afford to spend hours each day at the gym, hoping to get into better shape. Well, the good news is that you don't have to! The Promise Fat Loss & Fitness System is designed to maximize the time you spend exercising each day so you can attain the health and fitness you desire and still have time to focus on other important facets of your life.

Life isn't particularly enjoyable when you no longer fit into your clothes and when you feel tired throughout the day. When you have a negative self-image, and when you have to limit activities you would like to do, such as mountain bike riding, roller-blading and hiking through the wilderness. The quality of your life will be compromised.

Your health and fitness enable you to enjoy all the wonderful aspects of your life. I don't want you to think that you have to give up anything meaningful in your life to attain better health and fitness. When your health and fitness improves, everything becomes more enjoyable. You can do all the activities you've always wanted to do but were afraid to or not able to do for the reasons I mentioned above. As I mentioned in the beginning of the book, all the time you need to commit to is three hours or 1.6 percent of the entire week. Is that too much time to dedicate to improve the quality and duration of your life? Now is the time to start living!

Spend less time in the gym

Summary

- Use The Promise Fat Loss & Fitness System to make your workouts more efficient. Spend less of your valuable time at the gym.

- Increasing your health and fitness enables you to enjoy a more satisfying lifestyle.

- The Promise Fat Loss & Fitness System will enable you to experience all the activities you have always wanted to do.

Chapter XI

Continuing the same workout will result in— nothing!

Jim, the burnout

Jim called me for a consultation because he had heard from colleagues that I was helping people get into wonderful shape. Jim was a small business owner and, like many, he didn't live an active lifestyle. He was six feet tall and weighed 230 pounds. Jim's main goal was to feel better and look like he did when he was in college. Jim wanted to reduce his thirty-eight inch waist to thirty-four inches and be around 200 pounds of lean muscle tone.

Jim started off by stating, "Other fitness instructors had me lifting weights in the past and it didn't work. I got a little stronger, but I didn't get any leaner. Weight training is too monotonous and I'm burned out on weights." I was shocked. I knew from my experiences with hundreds of clients that weight training absolutely works. In fact, weight training is the only way to lose body fat and increase the metabolism permanently. I needed to know what Jim tried that did not work.

I asked him to describe his previous weight training routine. Jim said, "I would do a weight training circuit designed by a fitness instructor three times a week. It was a series of weight-bearing machines, probably around ten different ones, both upper body and lower body." I asked how many times he went through the circuit and he said twice each workout. I then asked him what else he did with weights and he said, "That's it."

I asked if the circuit or exercises ever changed and Jim said, "No. The instructor told me those ten machines hit all the major muscle groups." I asked him if he ever varied the weight or resistance of the machines and he said, "No." Then I asked Jim if he ever lifted free weights and once again the answer was "No." I finally asked Jim how long he had done that particular circuit and he said, "About eight weeks, then I just quit." I replied, "You know, you're right. If you do the same exercises with the same weights and in the same order three times a week you'll burn out and not get any results."

Jim looked confused and seemed a little bit stunned. I told him the circuit training he had performed was good for the first week of the program, but the circuit routine, the exercises and the resistance must change. I explained how muscle tissue is adaptive. If you don't constantly change the load or stimuli to the muscle, the muscle tissue won't have to adapt and change. Therefore, lean muscle tissue can't be developed, body fat won't decrease and results won't be attained. The body will get accustomed to anything done repeatedly.

I told Jim that working with resistance machines is all right, but working with free weights is much better. When you work with free weights, the body *must* balance the weight. Also, most people are either right side or left side dominant. Free weight training makes you use both sides equally. These two aspects of weight training challenge the muscle tissue better and produce more heat (burn more calories) than machine training. Boredom is also reduced with weight training because you must focus your attention on the exercise. The weight isn't on guide rods or cables so you have to be attentive. There's no time for boredom.

Jim said, "It sounds like it makes sense, but I don't know." I asked him to give my system a try. I PROMISED him that he wouldn't become bored with my system and that he would see wonderful results like his colleagues. Jim said, "All right, let's do it!"

I knew Jim would do well on my system, but he did better than I even imagined. He was a naturally big guy and was able to develop lean muscle quickly. In four months, he had achieved his thirty-four inch waist and his scale weight was a cool 197 pounds! Jim's body fat had dropped by seven percent in three months and he told me, "I feel better than when I was in college!"

Continuing the same workout will result in—nothing!

The body is amazingly adaptive. When it sheds fat due to changes in eating and activity, it is actually adapting to a new stimulus. Therefore, if you continue with the same workout every week, you will hit what exercisers refer to as a plateau. Your workout will no longer be new and your body will no longer have to adapt to a different stimulus. In fact, your body will get so conditioned to the same workout, it will actually *lose muscle tone and burn less fat* because it doesn't have to work as hard to attain the results. You may even get *fatter* during exercise!

In order to prevent the plateau from occurring, it is *essential* to modify and change your workout often. This is where a good personal trainer is valuable. "Periodization" is the term personal trainers use for workout variation. Without getting too scientific, if you constantly change the stimuli to your muscles through workload, intensity and exercise variation, your body will need to recruit different muscle tissues to meet this new challenge. The Promise Fat Loss & Fitness System provides the exercise variation that enhances the achievement of your fitness goals.

Because recruitment of different muscle tissue requires your body to perform in a way that is not customary, your muscle tissue will be constantly challenged. You will develop lean, toned muscle tissue.

Vary your workouts in order to tone muscle and lose fat.

if I lost you here—just remember that lean muscle tissue increases your metabolism and burns body fat. Workout variation is essential to this process. You can't perform the same exercises with the same weights and the same repetitions each workout and expect favorable results.

In The Promise Fat Loss & Fitness System our training guidelines include:

- Three weeks of circuit training that involves performing more repetitions with lighter weights.
- Three weeks of endurance training engaging in interval training with shortened rest periods.
- Three weeks of power strength training focusing on muscle growth.

If you don't understand the meaning of each of these workouts, don't be concerned at this point. This system will lead you step-by-step through the various exercise programs I have identified. The workouts have been designed to eliminate guesswork on your part; they will tell and show you exactly what exercises to perform, how many repetitions to do and when changes should be made. For additional help, our website, www.AlessiFit.com, demonstrates each exercise. Use this website to ensure you are performing them correctly.

If you are reading this book and are still unsure of how to begin the system, I strongly encourage you to schedule an appointment with a personal fitness professional. Even if you don't feel that having a trainer is right for you, a fitness consultation would be useful to get started. A fitness professional can help you define your goals and clarify how this system can help you achieve the success you desire. If you need additional help, contact my office where Don and I can conduct a telephone consultation.

Continuing the same workout will result in—nothing!

Summary

- If you don't change your workout often, you will plateau.

- When you plateau, you will either stay the same or get fatter.

- Following The Promise Fat Loss & Fitness System will constantly challenge your muscles to adapt to different stimuli by employing workout variation.

- If you are still unsure of how to complete this system, contact a fitness professional or my office for assistance.

Chapter XII

There is no such thing as the perfect time!

Dave: "I'll start fresh next week"

This is a story I regret to use as an example, for reasons you will soon understand. Dave was one of the first clients Don and I had worked with. He was in his early forties, overweight and a smoker. He was unathletic and new to exercise, but he wanted to improve his health and fitness. He knew he should take the time to change his unhealthy behaviors and improve his lifestyle.

Dave began his fitness program beautifully. He worked out hard and was beginning to eat better. Within a few weeks he had already lowered his scale weight seven pounds and increased his strength and endurance. He was looking better and, more importantly, feeling better. His body was his first priority.

Unfortunately, after six to eight weeks, Dave began to falter. He worked as a furniture dealer and often had to travel out of town to meet potential buyers. At first, Dave would only miss an occasional workout, but soon this number grew. Within a few months, he was missing workouts regularly. Don and I often spoke to him about recommitting to his body. We asked him, "Dave, you've already made progress and come so far. Do you really want to back track and start all over again?" He responded, "No, I don't want to give up progress, but I'm too busy this week. *I'll start fresh next week.*"

Don and I were new to the fitness business at that time and we believed Dave. We weren't as astute at seeing through excuses as we are now, and we expected him to recommit himself the following week. However, this setback had nothing to do with Dave being overly busy at work. He was making the same excuse millions of individuals do each day—he was procrastinating.

Whenever I hear anybody say, "I'm not going to work out today because I'm too busy" or "I don't feel good today; I'll work out tomorrow," I honestly believe they have good intentions. At the time, they believe they *will* work out later or tomorrow. However, this behavior is a mindset, not a scheduling problem. When you procrastinate or refuse to take action with your body, you're conditioning your mind to neglect your health and fitness. You're sending a mental signal that your body is not your top priority.

This is why it's so important to schedule your workouts and stick to your schedule. No time will ever be perfect and there will never be a better time than now. Another personal trainer and a colleague of mind once told me, "Derek, anyone can work out when they feel good. However, when you work out and don't feel 100 percent or don't have the time, then you'll make progress."

This inconsistent behavior went on for months. Dave put on the seven pounds he had lost plus an additional eight pounds. He lost his strength and his endurance. He felt physically awful and looked terrible, but he kept assuring Don and I that he would *start fresh next week.*

Finally, next week never came. Dave missed his Monday workout appointment. When Don called his house to see why he had missed, he learned that Dave had suffered a heart attack and died at age forty-three. Don and I were shocked.

I'm not telling you this story to scare you. I'm telling you what can happen if you don't make your health and fitness a priority. You, like Dave, are too young and have too much living left to do to allow this ill fate. I PROMISE you will never regret spending time on your body. But do it now—there is no such thing as the perfect time.

There is no such thing as the perfect time!

There is no such thing as the perfect time!

I've often heard prospective clients tell me the current time isn't good for them to begin a health and fitness program. Some of the most common rationalizations (excuses) I've heard include: "I'm too busy at work," "I have to check my schedule," "I'll begin after the holidays," "I want to wait until the kids are back in school," "I'll be traveling a lot over the next several months," or "I'm busy outdoors in the summer."

I PROMISE if you think long and hard enough you can probably come up with at least five reasons why you *cannot* begin a health and fitness program. In fact, this is exactly what most Americans do. They tell me or themselves *why* this isn't a good time to begin a healthy lifestyle. Consequently, this is the reason most Americans (sixty-one percent) are overweight or obese. They think everything in their lives must be perfect before they can begin a life improvement system. Unfortunately, no time will ever be perfect! *This is a dangerous mind set that you must avoid!*

You've procrastinated enough and your health and fitness levels have suffered. Every day you procrastinate is another day further from your goals, dreams and better health. Don't make the same mistake that millions of Americans do by convincing yourself that you can't exercise today. The time to do it is now! Even if you're tired; even if you have a mild cough or congestion; even if you have a busy day, do it today! There will never be a better time than now.

There is no such thing as the perfect time!

Summary

- Don't fool yourself into thinking you'll begin to work out tomorrow, next month or after the holidays. Do it now!

- Every day you procrastinate is another day further from your goals, dreams and better health.

- There is no such thing as the perfect time.

Part II
A New Life

Chapter XIII

Begin your transformation

I n the first three weeks of this system you will begin your transformation. The goal is to start to increase lean muscle tissue and get your metabolism moving. I don't want you to focus on your scale weight; rather, I want you to focus on your ability to burn fat and process food.

In this initial phase, you should learn to identify the real ingredients in foods and attempt to eat a supportive meal every three to three and a half hours. At first, if it is a challenge to eat every three hours, try to plan your meals in advance. When you get hungry, you'll eat whatever you can find if you haven't planned your meals. I suggest you plan meals for no less than one full day at a time. It's even better if you plan meals for the next two to three days in advance. Many of my private clients say this is the *single* biggest reason why they're able to eat well and reap the benefits of meal frequency and increased metabolism. I make it easy for my clients by having gourmet supportive meals available to them. A personal chef prepares these meals according to my criteria. The menu changes often and offers plain as well as exotic foods. They really have no excuse not to eat supportively!

Unfortunately, if you're expecting my brother Don or me to walk into your office with a hot plate of glazed turkey breast, sweet potatoes and lemon and herb green beans, you'd better not hold your breath! Seriously, though, if you have access to a refrigerator at work or if you can pack a small personal cooler, you have no excuse not to stick to the program. Please take the time to stock your refrigerator or cooler with supportive foods. Planning ahead really works and will accelerate your results.

Supplementation

A supplement is something that is used in addition to—not instead of—food. It's the "something extra." Many clients have asked me if a certain supplement is "worth it." I PROMISE if you are not eating supportive nutrition every three to three and a half hours, increasing your lean muscle tissue and performing a moderate amount of cardiovascular training, no supplement is "worth it." Supplements will *not* work by themselves. The following is a synopsis of various supplements.

Essential Fatty Acids

If you're adhering to The Promise Fat Loss & Fitness System, supplements will make the whole process more efficient. I strongly recommend consuming an essential fatty acid (EFA or omega-3 oils). Some of the best oils are flax, fish or hemp (it's not illegal!) Essential fatty acids help stabilize your blood sugar level, make your insulin receptors more efficient and satiate your body so you won't crave sugar. These oils are most effective in liquid, seed or ground forms rather than pills. My experience has shown that some people have trouble with the taste of the oil in liquid form. It's a "yuck" for them!

I suggest taking flax or hemp liquid with a chaser like a diet soda. It can also be blended into a protein shake, and some of my clients tell me they enjoy using it as a salad dressing. Personally, I mix ground flax seeds in my oatmeal every morning and add a scoop of protein powder (more on that later). This provides a complete breakfast and is an effective way to consume flax. Follow the serving size on the container. Don't cook with EFA oils because the properties will be changed and you won't get their benefits. Also available are flax seed crackers, made with 100 percent whole wheat and flax seeds. Use the crackers as a snack, not as a replacement for EFAs in liquid, ground or seed form.

EFAs are one of the best supplements to help you reach your goals of lowering your body fat and developing lean muscle tissue.

Post-Workout Protein Drinks

I recommend you consume a protein drink *immediately* after a weight training or cardiovascular training workout. On the days you perform both weight training and cardio, drink the protein shake at the end of the entire workout, not after each workout segment.

When you weight train, you create microscopic tears in muscle tissue. Remember, muscles are made of protein and protein is needed for muscle tissue to recuperate and repair itself. When muscle tissue is repaired, it becomes stronger and denser than it was initially, thus your body will develop muscle tissue. Consumption of post-workout protein helps this process.

A good protein supplement should be derived from a blend of whey, casein and egg protein. These types of protein promote the highest levels of protein assimilation (absorption into the body). If you're a strict vegetarian and don't wish to add protein sources from animal products, I suggest consuming soy protein powder. Though soy protein doesn't assimilate as well as a multi-blend of protein, it will help muscle tissue repair after weight training and is better than not consuming any protein post-workout.

Immediately after a weight training workout, your muscle cells are depleted of glycogen and best able to handle protein intake for their rebuilding. So as soon as you rack the weights, gulp a protein shake down! This will enhance development of your lean muscle tissue. Be sure to follow the serving size and directions on the package.

Many fitness professionals and scientists differ concerning the quantity of protein that can be absorbed at one time. I've read reports that suggest anywhere between twenty grams and 100 grams! Protein absorption will vary per individual based on size, amount of muscle tissue, age and activity level. While no one knows the exact protein absorbability, I personally suggest you consume a minimum of twenty-five grams in your post-workout shake. Contact a nutritionist if you have additional questions about protein consumption.

Meal Replacement Shakes

If you travel often and *don't* have access to a refrigerator or a cooler of food from home, I suggest you carry a meal replacement shake, which should consist of a balance of proteins, carbohydrates and some essential fats. Your muscles and your metabolism need this nourishment for development. The difference between a meal replacement shake and a protein shake is that a meal replacement shake is a "meal replacement." A protein shake does not contain carbohydrates or fats and is most effective immediately following a workout. A meal replacement shake can be consumed anytime in place of a meal.

I'm not suggesting if you don't travel that you cannot have or shouldn't have a meal replacement shake. You can absolutely have a meal replacement shake at home or the office. They can be an acceptable substitute for real food, especially if you're not going to eat otherwise. However, if you have the choice, *always* opt for real food. Also, make sure your meal replacement shake doesn't contain saturated fats and hydrogenated oils and has very few (less than three) grams of simple sugars per serving. Check out our website, www.AlessiFit.com, for a list of recommended meal replacement and protein shakes.

Protein Bars

Marketers are having a field day selling protein bars. They're found in most health food stores, grocery stores, department stores and even gas stations! Protein bars should be eaten only when you *do not* have access to real food. They're only useful in keeping your metabolism moving when you wouldn't eat otherwise. I predict that they will become less popular in the coming years when consumers discover the actual contents of the bars.

The nutritional content of protein bars is typically *not* what the manufacturer claims on the label. First, protein has a limited shelf life. If a label on a bar claims that it contains forty grams of protein, this means that it had forty grams of protein at the time it was manufactured. Often, it has much less protein by the time you eat it several months later.

Secondly, bar manufacturers often use a product called glycerin or glycerol as a sweetener. Glycerol is a sugar; however, it is an alcohol sugar. The Food and Drug Administration (FDA) doesn't require alcohol byproducts to be listed on food labels. So, manufacturers can claim their bar contains "zero carbohydrates," even when it's sweetened with glycerol or other simple sugars such as aorbitol, xylitol and mannitol. These sugars will react in your body the same way as sucrose or fructose. Thus you believe you're eating a supportive protein source when in actuality, you're eating a dry candy bar! Remember, you can always locate these sugars on the ingredients list.

Eat a protein bar as infrequently as possible. You won't get the nourishment your muscle tissue needs for development and the hidden sugar will sabotage your goals. A meal replacement shake is a better alternative than a protein bar for supportive nutrition. Always, real food is the best choice.

The importance of water

I recommend you drink a minimum of sixty-four ounces of water a day throughout the next eighteen weeks. If you don't know what sixty-four ounces is, get a sixteen-ounce water bottle, fill it up and drink it four times a day. Remember, if you want to speed up your metabolism, it's very important to develop lean muscle tissue. Since muscle tissue is roughly composed of eighty percent water, it behooves you to increase your water intake. The more water your muscles can hold, the more muscle you will have.

Any type of cell in your body needs only two elements to be healthy and grow: oxygen and water. If you nourish your cells properly, they will become healthier and stronger. In your muscle tissue, adequate water intake facilitates recuperation and development more efficiently and to a greater extent than is possible without adequate water intake.

Water also dilutes toxins in your body. If you recall from high school biology class, respiration occurs within your cells and results in the production of carbon dioxide. Water is fundamental in transporting carbon dioxide and other toxins away from the cells, thus assisting your blood in cell purification. Further, water helps muscle hydration, which in turn enhances muscle endurance.

A good rule to remember is that the more muscle tissue you have and the larger you are, the more water you should drink. Also,

Drink a minimum of sixty-four ounces of water a day. That is eight glasses, eight ounces each.

it's necessary to consume a generous amount of water after exercise to rehydrate your body. Your body will naturally lose water during a workout.

It's important not to drink too much water during your workout. Excess water will swish around in your stomach and make you feel sick, and can potentially lead to abdominal cramping. I've witnessed hundreds of individuals consume too much water during workouts, only to feel sluggish and sick. As I tell my clients, drink water sparingly during the workout and then *drink until you float* after the workout.

Please note: sixty-four ounces of water per day means pure water. Water contained in coffee, tea and soda or sugar-based drinks is *not* pure water! Most of these beverages will do more to dehydrate you than to adequately hydrate your body. I'm not saying that you cannot drink coffee or tea, just realize they don't count toward your desired water intake.

One last thought on water: unless you are an athlete or are competing in endurance events, please don't drink Gatorade or other sports drinks. I know the commercials for these products make you think their product is better than water because it replaces vitamins and minerals you excrete when working out. However, you probably won't lose that many vitamins and minerals during your workout. These drinks contain a very high concentration of simple sugars, which can turn to fat in your body. Water is a much better alternative to achieving your goal of decreasing body fat.

Protein Day

After you have conditioned your body to exercising and eating supportive nutrition for the first three weeks, I introduce a "protein day" into the system. The protein day is designed to accelerate the reduction of your body fat. I still want you to continue to eat every three to three and a half hours; however, you should *not* consume a slow-releasing carbohydrate on protein days. Instead, I want you to eat a larger serving (one and a half times the size of your fist) of protein and vegetables so your body doesn't undergo calorie deprivation.

On non-weight training days, your body will be forced to use fat for energy if the amount of sugar (both simple and complex) in your body is reduced. Don't eliminate slow-releasing complex carbohydrates on weight training days because your body will need them for sustained energy levels. Although vegetables contain complex carbohydrates, the high amount of fiber contained in vegetables is helpful in aiding body fat reduction and promotes satiation or "fullness."

Sometimes clients ask me about the amount of protein grams that should be consumed in a day. There's no easy way to answer this question. Overall, macronutrient consumption (protein, carbs or fats) depends upon fitness goals, body size, age and other health considerations. However, I want to remind you that lean protein is not calorically dense. For example, 100 grams of a lean protein source is equivalent to 400 calories. Most adults should be able to easily consume 400 calories of protein a day. If you want to simplify your life, forget all macronutrient grams and use your fist as a guide as I mentioned in Chapter IV. This way you will be eating a small amount of lean protein five times a day.

Fiber

Fiber is classified as either soluble or insoluble. Both types are important and necessary to a balanced and supportive nutrition plan.

Soluble fiber helps reduce cholesterol. Examples of soluble fiber are oats, oat bran, oatmeal, beans, peas and barley. Oats have a greater proportion of soluble fiber than any other grain.

Insoluble fiber is important in promoting normal bowel functions and digestion. Insoluble fiber includes whole-wheat breads, wheat cereals, wheat bran, rye and most other whole grains.

The American Heart Association (AHA) suggests eating a variety of foods to obtain fiber. The AHA in its medical article, "Fiber, Lipids, and Coronary Heart Disease," states, "Total dietary intake should be 25–30 grams a day (of fiber)." Further, the AHA suggests that it is desirable to "intake of both types of fiber in a ratio of one part soluble to three parts insoluble fiber."

Recent AHA findings indicate that fiber also reduces the risk of obesity: "It has been hypothesized that high-fiber foods may favorably impact satiety and slow gastric emptying, thereby sustaining a feeling of fullness that prohibits overeating. Intake of high-fiber foods may also improve glycemic control in diabetic individuals and reduce risk of insulin resistance." Other positive benefits of fiber include reducing low density lipoproteins (LDL, "bad" cholesterol) and blood pressure. Lastly, the AHA warns that, "Many commercial oat bran and wheat bran products (muffins, chips, waffles) actually contain very little bran." It's important to stay with foods like oatmeal (not packaged) and whole wheat bread.

In The Promise Fat Loss & Fitness System, you will eat foods high in both soluble and insoluble fiber. This will help you attain all of the above benefits. In addition to eating whole foods containing fiber, I also suggest you take an insoluble fiber supplement once a day. I recommend guar gum in either pill or powder form. Follow the directions on the label and consult with your physician if you have any questions. Another product new on the market is Satietrol®, manufactured by PacificHealth Laboratories. It contains guar gum, potato fiber and protein as well as other fibers into one package. Adequate fiber intake helps digestion, lowers cholesterol, blood pressure and your body fat.

Day's End

I'm often asked, "What time should I stop eating for the day?" Again, there is no easy answer. You must first consider your goals. If you want to lose body fat, I share the opinion of many other fitness professionals when I recommend you stop eating within three hours of bedtime. Your body doesn't need or use many calories while you are sleeping. So if you provide fuel for your body and perform no activity to utilize the fuel, your body will store it as fat.

If your goal is to increase muscle mass and size and you don't have a major concern with body fat reduction, it's advisable to eat a protein source before bedtime. This is because your body will break down protein and muscle tissue while you sleep. In order to prevent or slow down this protein cannibalization, you should consume some type of lean protein source, like cottage cheese, before bedtime. Remember, do this only if you are *not concerned* about losing body fat.

Chapter XIV

Questions and answers

Q: What if I don't have enough time to exercise?

A: I've heard this one for years. Well guess what—neither Don nor I have the time, either! I have a clientele that includes physicians, attorneys, financial planners, professors, CEOs and the mayor, and none of these people have the time to exercise. In fact, I've never had the privilege of hearing a client say to me, "Derek, I would really love to get into shape and I have all the time in the world. Could you train me and give me something to do to help me occupy my days?"

Probably, no one has the time to exercise and eat supportive meals frequently. However, human beings will make the time for things that they believe are important. If you're unwilling to make time for your health and fitness, they are clearly not your highest priority.

As I mentioned in earlier, I personally train many financially wealthy clients who have neglected their health to build their wealth and then attempt to use their wealth to buy back their health. Often they are unsuccessful at reversing the effects of obesity, diabetes, heart disease, osteoporosis and chronic fatigue. Every one of these clients tells me the same thing: "I wish I would have taken better care of my health and fitness sooner." This is a sad situation in which many individuals find themselves. Remember, no one ever said at the end of his or her life, "I wish I had spent more time at the office!"

Q: Am I too old?

A: No!—unless you're no longer moving, breathing or processing food. Don and I have worked with clients well into their late eighties! If they can do it, you can do it, too. As mentioned earlier, I advise you to check with your physician or health care professional before starting an exercise program, especially if you believe your health may be in question.

I do believe that your health and fitness goals should be consistent with your age. For example, I wouldn't begin a program designed to promote dramatic body fat reduction with someone who is eighty years old. However, I believe someone that age in good health can improve their lean muscle mass, strength and endurance. This will help them feel and move better, as well as increasing bone density. It's never too late to start.

Q: I've never stuck with an exercise program before. Am I doomed to fail?

A: You're only doomed if you believe that you are. Your mental attitude toward health and fitness is extremely important. If you believe you can follow this system, you will. If you believe you cannot follow this system or any other, you won't. Success or failure depends upon you.

I believe this system is more complete than most others. As I stated in the introduction, other "diets" you may have tried use an approach that couldn't possibly work for the long run. So, you didn't fail; the "diet" or "quick fix" plan failed you. Try The Promise Fat Loss & Fitness System, complete all the workouts and nutritional recommendations, and I PROMISE you great success in accomplishing your goals.

Q: I don't like to exercise. What else can I do?

A: I wish I could wave a magic wand and you could get all the benefits of exercise without ever having to break a sweat. In fact, marketers of many diet pills, electro-stimulation machines, ab rollers and infomercial gadgets know Americans want the easy way out and *prey* on it. They claim their product gives you all the benefits of exercise and proper nutrition without you ever having to lift a finger or change your behavior. These claims are misleading, deceptive and, in many cases, outright bogus. The goal of these phony products and gadgets is to make money. I think by now you know that improving your health and fitness by use of these products is impossible. The only thing that will be thinner after you purchase these products will be your wallet!

I know many of my clients don't like to exercise, but they do it and are committed to it because it helps them feel better and look better. They also value their health and want to prevent the occurrence of lifestyle-related diseases. I'm not asking you to quit your job and become a personal trainer, and I realize for some of you, exercise is not the pinnacle of your day. However, with a focused system and appropriate goals, I believe you may appreciate the value of exercise and do it even if it isn't your favorite thing. Your workouts will be challenging and changing constantly. The time you spend exercising will be effective and move you closer to your goals in an efficient manner.

Q: Am I too fat?

A: No! Don and I have helped dozens people to lose more than 100 pounds of fat and dramatically transform their life. We've seen hundreds of people lose more than fifty pounds of fat, increase their lean muscle mass and reduce their waistlines in half. You're never too fat to undertake a program to improve. However, I want you to realize the more fat you have, the longer it will take to accomplish your goals. But, as long as you are alive, there's still time to improve your health and fitness. I usually set a goal with my clients to reduce their body fat by two to four percent a month. This can be reasonably accomplished by following The Promise Fat Loss & Fitness System.

Q: I've tried other programs before and they didn't work. How is this one different?

A: As I said before, you didn't fail, miracle "diets" and fat loss products you may have tried failed *you*. By reading this far, you've learned how your body works. You now know that any system that doesn't contain steps for developing lean muscle tissue, supportive nutrition, and moderate cardiovascular training is incomplete and doomed to fail. My system includes all of these components necessary for success. This is the only complete system that ever took the time to educate you on how your body works.

Q: Will weight lifting make me look too bulky?

A: No. I know many women, and some men, are worried about becoming big and bulky. If you don't want to look big and bulky you need to lose body fat and develop your lean muscle tissue. Muscle tissue is lean and takes up almost four times less space than fat! A pound of fat takes up as much room as your clenched fist, whereas a pound of lean muscle tissue takes up as much room as a silver dollar. Unless you are into taking male hormones and steroids and spending four hours a day in the gym, there is *absolutely no way* you'll ever look like a body builder. Weight training and body fat reduction will make you appear lean and healthy.

Q: Why should I exercise if I can just take a pill that will increase my metabolism?

A: You need to be aware there is no such thing as a "magic pill" that will increase your metabolism. Remember, your metabolism is the rate at which your body processes and utilizes fuel. Only the development of lean muscle tissue, supportive nutrition and moderate cardiovascular training will increase the rate at which your body processes fuel. You may buy pills that claim they are metabolism enhancers, however, you will *only* increase your heart rate. These pills are *dangerous* and won't work for the long run, even if you lose water weight initially.

The reason you could initially lose weight with these pills is because your heart is a pump. If you increase the speed at which your heart pumps, it will extract more water out of your system, but this isn't the excess water that your body stores in your bladder. It is water located in your muscles, internal organs and cells.

You now know that your muscle tissue is composed of nearly eighty percent water, so if you decrease the water content in your muscle tissue, you'll have less muscle tissue. Less muscle tissue will lead to a slower metabolism. Consequently, taking pills you believe will increase your metabolism will actually have the opposite effect in the long run!

"Metabolism increasing" pills can also potentially be dangerous. They often have side effects that include dizziness, jitteriness, headaches and inability to concentrate. Increased pressure on your heart may also result from the ability of these pills to elevate blood pressure and speed heart rate. Since many of these pills contain "the stack," a mixture of caffeine, ephedrine and aspirin, they can be addictive.

Caffeine and ephedrine are stimulants; they will artificially increase your heart rate. Together they act as a small dosage of speed. Aspirin will thin your blood and increase the rate at which the stimulants enter your body. Since your goal is to increase your *health* and fitness, I would strongly recommend avoiding these products.

Q: Do fat blockers work to help reduce body fat and weight?

A: No! "Fat blockers" have not been proven to work in reducing body fat. The only thing they block is necessary, essential dietary fat from properly nourishing your body. Remember, consumption of dietary fat is not the only way a person gains weight. As you've learned through reading my system, you could become very fat even if you don't consume *any* dietary fat. If you consume excess sugar or even excess protein, your body will convert what you don't use to body fat.

Dietary fat and body fat aren't the same. Some types of unsaturated dietary fat are an essential macronutrient that you must consume to be healthy and for body processes to function normally. Body fat is the accumulation of excess adipose tissue, produced by your body's inability to utilize your ingestion of food.

If you use a *legitimate* "fat blocker" (obtained with a prescription, not through an infomercial!) you will most likely become deficient in essential fatty acids (dietary fat). When this happens, your body will break down muscle tissue to provide itself with essential fats and you will lose lean muscle tissue. This reduction of lean muscle tissue will slow down your metabolism and increase your body fat in the long run.

Further, many prescription fat blockers are associated with undesirable side effects, for example, changes in bowel habits, gas with discharge, an urgent need to go to the bathroom, oily or fatty stools, an oily discharge, increased number of bowel movements and an inability to control bowel movements. Unless you have a medical condition that warrants treatment from a physician, you should not take a fat blocker.

Q: What would happen if I just stop eating to lose weight?

A: You'll become fatter! If you stop eating, you'll lose water and lean muscle tissue. Muscle tissue is the only place in your body that burns fat and calories, so if you lose muscle, you'll slow down your body's ability to burn fat and calories. The initial decrease in your scale weight will soon be replaced by the addition of body fat and your metabolism will slow down. You'll condition yourself to be fatter, and you'll also be hungry and more apt to binge eat. Don't stop eating!

Q: I'm not sure I have the willpower to get in shape. How can I stick to this system?

A: You must *decide* to stick to this system. It's not a matter of will power; it's a matter of commitment. You must commit yourself to:

- Improving your health and fitness.
- Following and completing the system.
- Becoming the best you have ever been.

If you can't dedicate yourself to these goals, there isn't a program in existence that will help you.

If you are willing to dedicate yourself to and follow The Promise Fat Loss & Fitness System, I PROMISE you'll achieve better health and fitness than you ever imagined possible. A healthy and fit attitude often creates internal momentum that will enable you to achieve your health and fitness goals.

Q: Am I just predestined to be fat?

A: No! I don't doubt genetic factors may be involved at some level in the development of muscle or fatty tissue. Children who grow up with parents who are obese have a tendency to become obese themselves. Often, the obesity link between parents and children has to do more with poor parental role modeling and behavior than DNA. However, the genetic tendency to be overweight can be modified if you commit yourself to developing lean muscle tissue, eating supportive meals and performing cardiovascular training in moderation.

I tell my clients, "It isn't your genes that are making you out of shape and unhealthy; it's your behavior." After I adjust the eating and exercise behavior of my clients, they no longer regard their genes as an obstacle or an excuse. When you practice lifestyle modification by following my system, you'll be surprised at how little genetic differences actually matter.

Q: I don't want to compromise the quality of my life by worrying about not eating and drinking items that I enjoy. Despite this, I still want to get into better health and fitness. Is it possible?

A: Yes! When you engage in The Promise Fat Loss & Fitness System, you'll find you don't have to compromise the things you enjoy in your life. You've decided to take charge and live your life and this will create enjoyment. When you dedicate yourself to this system, you won't feel deprived; you'll feel proud of yourself for making the changes to improve your health and fitness.

You're an interesting and exciting person. You're so much more than junk food and alcohol. Don't believe that, with limiting your consumption of certain foods and beverages, life won't be worth living. Remember, you can have whatever you desire in moderation on your "cheat day." You'll feel and move better. You'll be able to do things that were physically impossible before. And you'll look better than you have in years. I PROMISE your quality of life will improve; it will not be compromised!

Q: I've read other books that tell me to "just love the real me" and not worry about my shape. How do you feel about that?

A: I believe that self-respect and self-confidence are extremely important. However, I don't think the premise of those books is to promote complacency and neglect your health and fitness. I believe they're trying to inform you that you don't have to look like a supermodel to feel worthy.

The Promise Fat Loss & Fitness System is based upon the theory that you can gain self-respect by improving your health and fitness while practicing an enjoyable lifestyle. Most individuals aren't aiming to be supermodels or professional athletes. This system is for regular people like you and me who have limited time each day to spend on health and fitness. It allows for achieving maximum health and fitness in an efficient manner.

Q: Why do I have to follow this system for eighteen weeks when I saw an advertisement that read "Lose thirty pounds in thirty days"? Is there a quicker way?

A: No! Remember, there are no short cuts to permanently lowering your body fat and fat weight. The advertisement you see on telephone poles or in commercials are usually promoting some "magic pill" that is supposed to increase your metabolism. As I said before, metabolism enhancers don't exist. Only weight training, supportive nutrition and moderate cardiovascular training will increase your metabolism. These magic pills will do no more than artificially raise your heart rate. In fact, ask yourself this question: "If these products worked so well, why wouldn't everyone who used them be in great shape?

The speed of your results depends on your goals and your fitness when you start the system. For example, if your goal is to lower your body fat two percent, you could probably accomplish this goal in one month. If you've never exercised before and you want to lose twenty percent body fat, seventy-five pounds of scale weight and drop six dress or suit sizes, You probably need to give yourself a reasonable timetable of at least twelve to fifteen months.

Q: Does liposuction work? If so, why can't I have it done instead of following this system?

A: Liposuction is a painful short-term surgical solution to a long-term behavioral problem. If you need a physician to suction fat out of your body with a vacuum, your health and fitness level will not be improved. You will have done nothing to improve your muscle tone, metabolism, strength, health, endurance, cardiovascular stamina and lifestyle behavior. In fact, most reputable plastic surgeons won't even perform this procedure on the casual individual looking to lose some fat.

Furthermore, you may look disproportionate. You can't have body fat removed from every site on your body simultaneously. You can have your tummy and hips done, but you may still have fat in your face, neck and back. Also, fat is a cell. Like all cells in your body, fat will divide and multiply.

If you give blood, you're not permanently short one pint of blood; your body will produce more blood cells. If you cut your hand, your body will produce more skin cells. If you have a tummy tuck and don't change the habits and lifestyle that led you to need the procedure, your body will produce more fat cells as well!

I recently read an advertisement for a group of plastic surgeons who were performing a free seminar for individuals interested in liposuction and "body contouring." The seminar discussed the process involved with the surgery. Reservations were required and refreshments of *wine, cheese and desserts* were served!

You need to treat the problem, not the short-term symptom. The Promise Fat Loss & Fitness System will teach you how to take control of your health and fitness for good. With this system, you'll learn how to lower your body fat permanently without having to go under the knife. And you'll improve so much more than just your appearance.

Q: Do women need a workout and nutritional program that is different from a man's?

A: Yes! However, the principles are the same. Both men and women need to learn to take control of their metabolism. Both need to develop lean muscle tissue, eat supportive meals frequently and perform a moderate amount of cardiovascular training.

In the ten years that I've been a personal fitness professional, I've learned women can't lift as much weight as men. (It really didn't take me that long to realize it!) Also, a woman should consume fewer calories than a man because she has a smaller amount of lean muscle tissue. However, the principles in The Promise Fat Loss & Fitness System apply equally to both men and women.

Q: How can I consult with you or Don for health and fitness advice?

A: Both Don and I work in our private training facilities in the Buffalo New York area. You can call our office, e-mail or write. We conduct telephone as well as in-office consultations, and we also specialize in corporate seminars.

Derek Alessi	Don Alessi
7662 Transit Road	300 Delaware Avenue
Williamsville NY 14221	Buffalo NY 14202
(716) 635-0758	(716) 853-4930
ThePromise@adelphia.net	D_Strength@hotmail.com

Chapter XV

Words of encouragement

I've enjoyed furthering your education about health, fitness and how your body works. I trust you found this book informative and motivational. As I mentioned at the beginning of this book, it doesn't matter if you are male or female. It doesn't matter if you are eighteen or eighty years old. It doesn't matter if you have ever been in shape before or ever stuck with an organized exercise plan for more than the two weeks after a New Year's resolution. You *have* the power to transform your health and fitness. As a result, you'll benefit from increased energy and productivity. You'll also be able to wear clothes that reveal your new shape. Most importantly, remember you have the power to increase your enjoyment of life!

You've learned how to take control of your nutritional habits and not be deceived by misleading food marketers, and gained understanding of the fraud behind fitness claims and radical diets. I have confidence you now have the basic tools you need to empower yourself and take control of your body. I'm also confident you've increased your self-confidence, self-respect and sense of personal empowerment through adhering to my 100 percent effective Promise System.

If this is the first time you've been exposed to this information, I encourage you to read it again or call for a personal fitness consultation. Don and I look forward to helping anyone who is serious about improving his or her health and fitness. Please don't hesitate to call our offices and tell us how you're doing with the system. Are you ready to begin?

As I said earlier, *do not* begin this program unless you are absolutely committed to:

- Improving your health and fitness.
- Following and completing the system.
- Becoming the best you have ever been.

Once you've done this, you'll attain every fitness goal you set out to accomplish. You'll look and feel the way you desire. You will have transformed your health and fitness!

On the following pages I have outlined my plan for the next 126 days. Follow these steps as if you were following a treasure map that leads you to gold.

You'll be beginning a new exercise program. Included are pictures and descriptions of exercises, as well as the workouts themselves. Remember, always use weight that you can handle. It's better to start light and increase weight as needed, than to use weights you can't handle and do it wrong. Our website, www.AlessiFit.com, visually demonstrates with streaming video how to perform the all exercises properly. If you have any questions about the workouts or exercises, please contact a personal fitness professional.

I'm going to ask you to do some additional cardiovascular training on some of your non-weight training days. On these days, it's important to do your cardio at a moderate pace. I define a moderate pace as being a level six or seven out of ten, with ten being the most difficult. Please don't go too fast or exceed the time I recommend. Remember, I don't want you to mentally burn out or break down muscle tissue.

I'm also going to ask you to rate your performance each day on a scale from one to ten, with one being the least effort you could possibly imagine and ten being your maximal effort. I don't expect you to be perfect every day; I know you're human. However, I want you to be as conscientious as possible. You need an honest evaluation of your effort for your own feedback. Your results will always parallel your effort. If you perform at a high rate for the day and the week, I PROMISE it will show in the results.

It's very important to rate yourself honestly. It won't help you if you give yourself a higher score than you deserve. So rate yourself honestly and accurately. I PROMISE your good effort will shine through!

I can only educate you so much—now it's time for you to execute the PROMISE. Good luck and stay committed to the plan. Your results depend upon it!

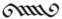

Promise Summary

- If you want to reduce your body fat for the rest of your life, never diet again.

- When you "diet" you condition your body to burn less fat and fewer calories.

- SYNERGY is the only way to permanently increase your metabolism.

- SYNERGY involves 1) developing lean muscle tissue 2) increasing the frequency of eating supportive meals and 3) performing a moderate amount of cardiovascular exercise.

- When you develop lean muscle tissue, you produce heat, which has a metabolic effect of burning fat and calories

- The more lean muscle tissue you have, the faster your metabolism will work.

- Lean muscle tissue takes up four times less space than fatty tissue.

- Eat a supportive meal every three to three and a half hours.

- The more frequently you eat, the more conditioned and efficient your body will become to burning food.

- A supportive meal contains a lean protein, a slow-releasing carbohydrate, and a vegetable (preferably green).

- Proteins are essential and provide twice as much thermal effect as carbohydrates or fats.

- Protein is necessary for the development of lean muscle tissue and ridding the body of fat.

- Incorporate one "cheat day" into your supportive eating habits.

- On your cheat day, eat whatever you want, in moderation.

- The body requires essential fatty acids (EFAs) such as flax, fish, and hemp oils, not saturated fats and hydrogenated oils.

- One gram of fat contains nine calories!

- Sugar causes an insulin response that ultimately leads to fat gain.

- Always check the ingredients list of foods so that you are less likely to be deceived by slick marketers.

- Consume no more than two servings of alcohol per week.

- Fruit is a simple sugar, so limit your consumption.

- Look at product labels to see if manufacturers are "sneaking" fats and sugars into the ingredients lists

- Consuming too much sugar or fat will increase your body fat and jeopardize your health and fitness goals.

- Performing too much cardiovascular training may break down your muscle tissue. This will slow down your metabolism and make you fatter.

- Spend less time doing cardiovascular training and more time engaging in weight training.

- Contact a personal fitness professional if you have questions regarding weight training or cardiovascular training workouts.

- If you don't change your workout often, you will plateau.

- Following The Promise Fat Loss & Fitness System will constantly challenge your muscles to adapt to different stimuli by employing workout variation.

- Don't fool yourself into thinking you'll begin to work out tomorrow, next month or after the holidays. Do it now!

- Every day you procrastinate is another day further from your goals, dreams and better health.

- There is no such thing as the perfect time!

There is nothing training cannot do.
Nothing is above its reach.
It can turn bad morals to good;
it can destroy bad principles
and recreate good ones;
it can lift men to angelship.

—Mark Twain

Part III
Time to Eat

Chapter XVI

Sample meal plans and grocery list

The following chart shows a sample day of supportive nutrition. If you have any questions regarding these meals or types of foods, consult with a nutritionist or dietician in your area.

You will notice meals are spaced three hours apart. It is essential you eat every three to three and a half hours to speed up your metabolism. Substitute any protein, slow-releasing carbohydrate and vegetable with any item listed on the second chart of supportive foods.

Sample Day of Supportive Nutrition

7 a.m.	Breakfast	Egg white omelet with wheat toast, flax seeds, guar gum fiber.
10 a.m.	Snack	Cottage cheese (1%) and whole wheat crackers
1 p.m.	Lunch	Grilled chicken over a bed of leafy lettuce, veggies and a sweet potato
4 p.m.	Snack	Meal replacement shake
7 p.m.	Dinner	Chicken/steak/fish with brown rice and veggies

Next, here is a list of some of the most common supportive foods:

Supportive Foods

Lean proteins	Slow-releasing carbohydrates	Vegetables
Egg whites	Wheat bread	Broccoli
Egg Beaters	Wheat pasta	Spinach
Chicken breast	Sweet potatoes/yams	Green beans
Turkey breast	Oatmeal	Asparagus
Steak	Brown rice	Mushrooms
Fish	Wild rice	Cauliflower
Shellfish	Whole grain couscous	Leafy lettuce
Cottage cheese (1%)		Peppers
Ostrich		
Pork		
Veal		
Buffalo (not the city)		
Tuna		
Protein powders		
Tofu		

Note: foods can be substituted

Quick and easy meal suggestions

Below I have included samples of my own supportive nutrition meals that can be used as a guide. I know you don't have a lot of time to plan your nutrition, so I'm not going to give you elaborate recipes that call for dozens of ingredients and several measuring cups. These are supportive meal combinations that can be prepared easily.

Derek's favorites

I usually wake up at 4:45 a.m. and make sure I eat a supportive breakfast (even though I'm half asleep!). The meals I suggest should take less than four minutes to prepare. If you still think you don't have time in the morning to eat breakfast, then wake up four minutes earlier! Remember, if you skip breakfast you'll slow down your metabolism and compromise your results. Make it a rule to *never* skip breakfast! The serving sizes below are for me. To customize this list for you, remember to use your clenched fist as a guide.

Breakfast

- Three egg whites with one whole egg or one carton of Egg Beaters
  One or two pieces of 100 percent whole or stone wheat bread
  Low fat cheese
  Cottage cheese (1%)

- Oatmeal (whole oats, not instant)
  One scoop protein powder
  Two tablespoons of ground flax seeds (as directed on container)

- Two pieces 100 percent whole or stone ground wheat toast
  Three tablespoons of cottage cheese (1%)

- Meal replacement shake
  Mix with two tablespoons of ground flax seeds (as directed on container)

Snack between breakfast and lunch or lunch and dinner

- Cottage cheese (1%) with 100 percent whole wheat or flax seed crackers

- Meal replacement shake

- Oatmeal with protein powder

- Egg Beaters (Can be prepared in a microwave at home or work)

- Apple with one tablespoon of peanut butter (no more than once per week)

- Sugar-free Jell-O or pudding

Lunch

- Green leafy salad with chicken or tuna. Add cucumbers, tomatoes and cheese for more taste. Use mixture of extra virgin olive oil with flax seed oil (preferred) or some type of reduced calorie dressing

- Chicken, turkey, or fish with brown rice or sweet potato and a green vegetable

- Chicken, turkey, or fish sandwich. Use 100 percent whole or stone ground wheat bread. Add hot sauce, mustard or reduced calorie salad dressing for flavor

- Chicken or tuna roll-ups. Roll strips of chicken or tuna fish in 100 percent whole wheat tortilla shells. Add low-fat cheese, a tomato and a small amount of mayonnaise (light) for taste

- Chicken or Steak Burrito (make yourself—don't buy from a fast-food restaurant!). Chicken or steak strips, low calorie cheese, leafy lettuce, tomato and salsa or hot sauce and whole wheat tortilla shells

Dinner
(Be careful not to overeat)

- Green leafy salad with chicken or tuna. Add cucumbers, tomatoes and cheese for more taste. Use mixture of extra virgin olive oil with flax seed oil (preferred) or some type of reduced calorie dressing

- Chicken, turkey, or steak with brown rice or sweet potato and a green vegetable

- Shrimp and chicken kabobs with green peppers, tomatoes and mushrooms

- White fish (orange roughy, haddock or sole) and a sweet potato, grilled

- Ground chicken, turkey or mixed poultry. Add taco seasoning over bed of brown rice or whole grain couscous, or include a whole wheat tortilla and green vegetable

- Steak filet and a sweet potato or whole grain couscous

Promise Grocery List

DAIRY
- ❑ Eggs/Egg Beaters
- ❑ Skim milk
- ❑ Butter
- ❑ Fat free plain yogurt
- ❑ Cottage cheese (1%)
- ❑ Tofu
- ❑ Low fat cheese

MEAT, FISH, POULTRY
- ❑ Chicken (ground or whole)
- ❑ Turkey (ground or whole)
- ❑ Beef
- ❑ Pork
- ❑ Ham (occasionally)
- ❑ Fish (as often as possible)
- ❑ Shellfish
- ❑ Bacon (cheat day)
- ❑ Sausage (lean)

FRUIT (cheat day)
- ❑ Berries
- ❑ Lemons
- ❑ Limes
- ❑ Oranges
- ❑ Pears
- ❑ Melon
- ❑ Apples

VEGETABLES
- ❑ Broccoli
- ❑ Green beans
- ❑ Cauliflower
- ❑ Celery
- ❑ Cucumbers
- ❑ Garlic
- ❑ Lettuce (leafy)
- ❑ Mushrooms
- ❑ Onions
- ❑ Peppers
- ❑ Sweet potatoes (yams)
- ❑ Spinach
- ❑ Tomatoes
- ❑ Asparagus

BREADS
- ❑ 100% Whole or Stone ground Wheat Bread
- ❑ 100% Whole Wheat Pitas or Tortillas

DRY GOODS
- ❑ Oatmeal (whole oats, not instant)
- ❑ Pasta (whole wheat)
- ❑ Beans, lentils or peas
- ❑ Rice (brown or wild)
- ❑ 100% whole or stone ground wheat crackers
- ❑ Flax crackers

CANNED GOODS
- ❑ Mushrooms
- ❑ Stewed Tomatoes
- ❑ Tuna (white albacore in water)
- ❑ Chicken (in water)

CONDIMENTS
- ❑ Extra virgin olive oil
- ❑ Mayonnaise (low fat)
- ❑ Mustard
- ❑ Relish
- ❑ Salsa
- ❑ Salad dressing (low fat)
- ❑ Hot sauce
- ❑ Peanut butter (reduced sugar/fat)

BEVERAGES
- ❑ Coffee
- ❑ Tea
- ❑ Soft drinks (sugar free)
- ❑ Crystal Light
- ❑ Bottled water
- ❑ Beer (cheat days)
- ❑ Wine (cheat days)

SUPPLEMENTS
- ❑ Protein powder (post-workout shake)
- ❑ Meal replacement shakes
- ❑ Flax seeds or oil/fish oil/hemp oil
- ❑ Fiber (guar gum or Satietrol®)

Part IV
Body in Motion

Anatomy of Major Muscle Groups

Shoulders
(Deltoids)

Arm
(Bicep)

Abs/Torso
(Obliques)

Quadricep
(Vastus lateralis)
outside muscle

Trapezius

Forearm
(Brachioradialis)

Abs/Torso
(Rectus abdominus)

Quadricep
(Vastus medialis)
inside muscle of quad

Back
(Infraspinatus)

Back
(Latissimus dorsi)

Glutes
(Gluteus maximus)

Back thigh
(Hamstrings)

Shoulders
(Deltoids)

Arm
(Tricep)

Back
(Erector spinae)

Calves
(Gastrocnemius)

These primary muscle groups are the focus of The Promise Fat Loss & Fitness System workouts.

115

Chapter XVII

Exercise instructions

The following workouts are designed to aid you in beginning a weight-training program. Use the next three sections—The Workouts, A Visual Guide to the Exercises, and Chart Your Progress—in unison. There is nothing "magical" about this or any other workout. You don't need to use this workout program if a personal trainer or some other qualified fitness professional has designed a workout for you. However, I do want you to follow my system of performing three weeks of circuit training, three weeks of endurance training and three weeks of power strength training. Remember, workout variation is absolutely necessary. Also, regardless of the type of resistance training you're doing, I want you to follow my nutritional and cardiovascular advice.

Circuit Training, weeks 1–3

For the first three weeks of the resistance workout, you're going to perform circuit training. Circuit training means that exercises are performed consecutively with little rest between. This is to get the metabolism moving and develop lean muscle tissue. For example, in workout one on page 172, you would begin with the warm-ups located inside the individual boxes at the left. Perform each warm-up once and hold for twenty seconds. Then perform exercise one, then two, then three, then four, then five, then six. That is set one and a complete circuit. You would then rest for two minutes and perform set two, the same circuit again. Depending on how you feel, you could perform the circuit a total of four times. Write your weights and repetitions under the picture. If necessary, change weight resistance for the exercise(s) before beginning next circuit.

You will notice cardiovascular suggestions below the workout chart. For example, in workout one, the cardiovascular suggestion is to perform fifteen minutes at level five exertion. You can use the treadmill, bike, stair stepper, elliptical machine or walk briskly outside. Don't exceed fifteen minutes to start. Remember, you don't want to exercise away valuable lean muscle tissue. As far as exertion or difficulty of cardiovascular training, perform at mid-level difficult. For example, level one would be extremely easy and level ten would be very difficult. Level five means at a good pace, but not too fast. I also recommend that you change your cardiovascular machine often. Don't always use the treadmill or any other machine. For example, walk on the treadmill on Tuesday, ride the stationary bike on Thursday and use the stair stepper on Saturday.

Endurance Training, weeks 4–6

In the fourth week, you will switch to endurance training. Endurance is different than circuit training in that an "endurance interval" is performed twice a set. For example, in workout ten on page 175, you will once again start with the warm-up, then perform exercise one, the bench press, followed by exercise two, dumbbell chest flys. Exercise three is the endurance interval which can include jump rope, bike, elliptical climber or running. Right after the interval, you would immediately begin exercise four and five, then the second interval. The endurance interval should be performed at a fast pace for the time allotted, which in workout ten is thirty seconds. The endurance interval is designed to spike your heart rate and condition your body to increase its endurance. Also, your body will produce additional lactic acid as a byproduct of the endurance interval. The additional lactic acid has a metabolic (calorie-burning) effect. So the endurance-training phase focuses on burning fat. After the first circuit or set, rest two minutes and repeat.

If you feel out of breath or light-headed, rest for a longer time or stop. Depending on your fitness level, endurance training may be difficult on your body.

Power Strength Training, weeks 7–9

In week seven on page 178, you will begin power strength training. This phase is designed to increase your strength and lean muscle tissue. Utilizing big muscle groups and performing multi-joint movements, you will create the most amount of heat in the muscle. You will also develop the most amount of lean muscle tissue in this phase. I'm often asked, "Derek, if this phase develops the most lean muscle tissue and burns the most fat, why don't we do it all the time?" The answer is that every workout routine needs to be constantly changed or muscle tissues will no longer be stimulated. Secondly, training too long with multi-joint exercises at a heavy weight and low repetitions can lead to injury. Therefore, you will only perform the power strength-training phase for three weeks at a time. Remember to start with the warm up. When performing power strength training, give yourself one and a half to two minutes between each exercise. Even though the focus of this phase is heavier weight with fewer repetitions, I advise you to start light and add weight as you feel the need to challenge yourself. Utilize www.Alessifit.com for a demonstration of these exercises. Also, this is the phase where a personal trainer will be most valuable. The power strength training exercises are the most difficult to perform and take the longest to learn. A trainer can help you learn these exercises safely and correctly.

After power strength training, the focus of the workout repeats back to circuit training. This time, focus on working the muscles more intensely by adding additional weight or repetitions.

- Weeks 10–12: Circuit training
- Weeks 13–15: Endurance training
- Weeks 16–18: Power strength training

Remember, these workouts are suggestions. I don't want you to get frustrated if these exercises are not available to you or if you find them difficult. If you are discouraged or are having trouble with any part of weight training, please contact a personal trainer for assistance. Don't quit—your results depend upon it!

Chapter XVIII

The Workouts

Week 1

If your workouts get off schedule from what is on the "game plan," just make sure that you're weight training three times per week and doing cardiovascular training six times per week. Refer to chapter XX to chart your progress and follow the circuit training workout.

Day 1: Circuit training: designed to begin to build lean muscle tissue and get the metabolism moving. You will also perform fifteen minutes of cardiovascular training.

EAT: Lean protein, slow-releasing carbohydrate, and vegetable every three to three and a half hours. Drink a minimum of sixty-four ounces of water and take a fiber supplement. Drink a meal replacement shake if necessary (if you won't eat otherwise).

Grade 1-10

Day 2: Ten minutes of cardiovascular training on your own. Make sure that you're moving at a moderate pace (about a level of six to seven on a scale of one to ten). You can walk, bike, stair step, cross-country ski or do any activity where you are moving continuously for at least ten minutes.

EAT: Lean protein, slow-releasing carbohydrate, and vegetable every three to three and a half hours. Drink a minimum of sixty-four ounces of water and take a fiber supplement. Drink a meal replacement shake if necessary.

Grade 1-10 ☐

Day 3: Circuit training: designed to begin to build lean muscle tissue and get the metabolism moving. You will also perform fifteen minutes of cardiovascular training.

EAT: Lean protein, slow-releasing carbohydrate, and vegetable every three to three and a half hours. Drink a minimum of sixty-four ounces of water and take a fiber supplement. Drink a meal replacement shake if necessary.

Grade 1-10 ☐

Day 4: Ten minutes of cardiovascular training on your own. Make sure that you're moving at a moderate pace.

EAT: Lean protein, slow-releasing carbohydrate, and vegetable every three to three and a half hours. Drink a minimum of sixty-four ounces of water and take a fiber supplement. Drink a meal replacement shake if necessary.

Grade 1-10 ☐

Day 5: Circuit training: designed to begin to build lean muscle tissue and get the metabolism moving. You will also perform fifteen minutes of cardiovascular training.

EAT: Lean protein, slow-releasing carbohydrate, and vegetable every three to three and a half hours. Drink a minimum of sixty-four ounces of water and take a fiber supplement. Drink a meal replacement shake if necessary.

Grade 1-10 ☐

Day 6: Ten minutes of cardiovascular training on your own. Make sure that you're moving at a moderate pace.

EAT: Lean protein, slow-releasing carbohydrate, and vegetable every three to three and a half hours. Drink a minimum of sixty-four ounces of water and take a fiber supplement. Drink a meal replacement shake if necessary.

Grade 1-10

Day 7: Rest, Cheat Day—Eat whatever you want, in moderation. Remember meal frequency!

Total Score for the Week

The total score for the week should not be less than 48. If it is, your effort will need to improve to see results!

Week 2

You'll progress with weight training to stimulate an increase in your metabolism and will begin to initiate some shifts in your percentage of body fat.

Day 8: Circuit training: designed to build lean muscle tissue and get the metabolism moving. You will also perform twenty minutes of cardiovascular training.

EAT: Lean protein, slow-releasing carbohydrate, and vegetable every three to three and a half hours. Drink a minimum of sixty-four ounces of water and take a fiber supplement. Drink a meal replacement shake if necessary.

Grade 1-10

Day 9: Fifteen minutes of cardiovascular training on your own. Make sure that you are moving at a moderate pace.

EAT: Lean protein, slow-releasing carbohydrate, and vegetable every three to three and a half hours. Drink a minimum of sixty-four ounces of water and take a fiber supplement. Drink a meal replacement shake if necessary.

Grade 1-10

Day 10: Circuit training: designed to build lean muscle tissue and get the metabolism moving. You will also perform twenty minutes of cardiovascular training.

EAT: Lean protein, slow-releasing carbohydrate, and vegetable every three to three and a half hours. Drink a minimum of sixty-four ounces of water and take a fiber supplement. Drink a meal replacement shake if necessary.

Grade 1-10

Day 11: Fifteen minutes of cardiovascular training on your own. Make sure that you are moving at a moderate pace.

EAT: Lean protein, slow-releasing carbohydrate, and vegetable every three to three and a half hours. Drink a minimum of sixty-four ounces of water and take a fiber supplement. Drink a meal replacement shake if necessary.

Grade 1-10

Day 12: Circuit training: designed to build lean muscle tissue and get the metabolism moving. You will also perform twenty minutes of cardiovascular training.

EAT: Lean protein, slow-releasing carbohydrate, and vegetable every three to three and a half hours. Drink a minimum of sixty-four ounces of water and take a fiber supplement. Drink a meal replacement shake if necessary.

Grade 1-10

Day 13: Fifteen minutes of cardiovascular training on your own. Make sure that you are moving at a moderate pace.

EAT: Lean protein, slow-releasing carbohydrate, and vegetable every three to three and a half hours. Drink a minimum of sixty-four ounces of water and take a fiber supplement. Drink a meal replacement shake if necessary.

Grade 1-10

Day 14: Rest, Cheat Day—Eat whatever you want, in moderation. Remember meal frequency!

Total Score for the Week ☐

Make sure your score is accurate! You will soon begin to see and feel results.

Week 3

You will once again increase the intensity of your weight training and cardiovascular training. By now, you should be getting conditioned to eating supportively.

Day 15: Last week of circuit training: designed to build lean muscle tissue and get the metabolism moving. You will also perform twenty-five minutes of cardiovascular training.

EAT: Lean protein, slow-releasing carbohydrate, and vegetable every three to three and a half hours. Drink a minimum of sixty-four ounces of water and take a fiber supplement. Drink a meal replacement shake if necessary.

Grade 1-10 ☐

Day 16: Twenty minutes of cardiovascular training on your own. Make sure that you are moving at a moderate pace.

EAT: Lean protein, slow-releasing carbohydrate, and vegetable every three to three and a half hours. Drink a minimum of sixty-four ounces of water and take a fiber supplement. Drink a meal replacement shake if necessary.

Grade 1-10 ☐

Day 17: Circuit training: designed to build lean muscle tissue and get the metabolism moving. You will also perform twenty-five minutes of cardiovascular training.

EAT: Lean protein, slow-releasing carbohydrate, and vegetable every three to three and a half hours. Drink a minimum of sixty-four

ounces of water and take a fiber supplement. Drink a meal replacement shake if necessary.

Grade 1-10 [　　]

Day 18: Twenty minutes of cardiovascular training on your own. Make sure that you are moving at a moderate pace.

EAT: Lean protein, slow-releasing carbohydrate, and vegetable every three to three and a half hours. Drink a minimum of sixty-four ounces of water and take a fiber supplement. Drink a meal replacement shake if necessary.

Grade 1-10 [　　]

Day 19: Last week of circuit training: designed to build lean muscle tissue and get the metabolism moving. You will also perform twenty-five minutes of cardiovascular training.

EAT: Lean protein, slow-releasing carbohydrate, and vegetable every three to three and a half hours. Drink a minimum of sixty-four ounces of water and take a fiber supplement. Drink a meal replacement shake if necessary.

Grade 1-10 [　　]

Day 20: Twenty minutes of cardiovascular training on your own. Make sure that you are moving at a moderate pace.

EAT: Lean protein, slow-releasing carbohydrate, and vegetable every three to three and a half hours. Drink a minimum of sixty-four ounces of water and take a fiber supplement. Drink a meal replacement shake if necessary.

Grade 1-10 [　　]

Day 21: Rest, Cheat Day—Eat whatever you want, in moderation. Remember meal frequency!

Total Score for the Week [　　]

Congratulations! You've made it through the first segment, but don't get on the scale yet! Next we begin endurance training.

Week 4

You will begin endurance training with shortened rest periods. This is designed to keep your heart rate elevated throughout the entire workout. New exercises are added and so is a protein day.

Day 22: Endurance training. Continue to build muscle and get the heart rate moving, baby! You will also perform thirty minutes of cardiovascular training.

EAT: Lean protein, slow-releasing carbohydrate, and vegetable every three to three and a half hours. Drink a minimum of sixty-four ounces of water and take a fiber supplement. Drink a meal replacement shake if necessary.

Grade 1-10

Day 23: Twenty minutes of cardiovascular training on your own. Make sure that you are moving at a moderate pace.

EAT: Protein Day. Lean protein and a vegetable every three to three and a half hours. Consume a minimum of sixty-four ounces of water and take a fiber supplement. To accelerate fat loss, don't eat carbohydrates on non-weight training days. Eat a larger portion of lean protein and vegetables. Drink a meal replacement shake if necessary.

Grade 1-10

Day 24: Endurance training. Continue to build muscle and get the heart rate moving. You will also perform thirty minutes of cardiovascular training.

EAT: Lean protein, slow-releasing carbohydrate, and vegetable every three to three and a half hours. Drink a minimum of sixty-four ounces of water and take a fiber supplement. Drink a meal replacement shake if necessary.

Grade 1-10

Day 25: Twenty minutes of cardiovascular training on your own. Make sure that you are moving at a moderate pace.

EAT: Protein Day. Lean protein and a vegetable every three to three and a half hours. Consume a minimum of sixty-four ounces of water and take a fiber supplement. Drink a meal replacement shake if necessary.

Grade 1-10 ▢

Day 26: Endurance training. Continue to build muscle and get the heart rate moving. You will also perform thirty minutes of cardiovascular training.

EAT: Lean protein, slow-releasing carbohydrate, and vegetable every three to three and a half hours. Drink a minimum of sixty-four ounces of water and take a fiber supplement. Drink a meal replacement shake if necessary.

Grade 1-10 ▢

Day 27: Twenty minutes of cardiovascular training on your own. Make sure that you are moving at a moderate pace.

EAT: Protein Day. Lean protein and a vegetable every three to three and a half hours. Consume a minimum of sixty-four ounces of water and take a fiber supplement. Drink a meal replacement shake if necessary.

Grade 1-10 ▢

Day 28: Rest, Cheat Day—Eat whatever you want, in moderation. Remember meal frequency!

Total Score for the Week ▢

You should begin to notice a change in the way your clothes fit. You're losing fat!

Week 5

You will continue endurance training with shortened rest periods. This is designed to keep your heart rate elevated throughout the entire workout.

Day 29: Endurance training. Continue to build muscle and get the heart rate moving. Also, perform thirty minutes of cardiovascular training.

EAT: Lean protein, slow-releasing carbohydrate, and vegetable every three to three and a half hours. Drink a minimum of sixty-four ounces of water and take a fiber supplement. Drink a meal replacement shake if necessary.

Grade 1-10 ☐

Day 30: Twenty minutes of cardiovascular training on your own. Make sure that you are moving at a moderate pace.

EAT: Protein Day. Lean protein and a vegetable every three to three and a half hours. Consume a minimum of sixty-four ounces of water and take a fiber supplement. To accelerate fat loss, don't eat carbohydrates on non-weight training days. Eat a larger portion of lean protein and vegetables. Drink a meal replacement shake if necessary.

Grade 1-10 ☐

Day 31: Endurance training. Continue to build muscle and get the heart rate moving. Also, perform thirty minutes of cardiovascular training.

EAT: Lean protein, slow-releasing carbohydrate, and vegetable every three to three and a half hours. Drink a minimum of sixty-four ounces of water and take a fiber supplement. Drink a meal replacement shake if necessary.

Grade 1-10 ☐

Day 32: Twenty minutes of cardiovascular training on your own. Make sure that you are moving at a moderate pace.

EAT: Protein Day. Lean protein and a vegetable every three to three and a half hours. Consume a minimum of sixty-four ounces of water and take a fiber supplement. Drink a meal replacement shake if necessary.

Grade 1-10 ☐

Day 33: Endurance training. Continue to build muscle and get the heart rate moving. Also, perform thirty minutes of cardiovascular training.

EAT: Lean protein, slow-releasing carbohydrate, and vegetable every three to three and a half hours. Drink a minimum of sixty-four ounces of water and take a fiber supplement. Drink a meal replacement shake if necessary.

Grade 1-10

Day 34: Twenty minutes of cardiovascular training on your own. Make sure that you are moving at a moderate pace.

EAT: Protein Day. Lean protein and a vegetable every three to three and a half hours. Consume a minimum of sixty-four ounces of water and take a fiber supplement. Drink a meal replacement shake if necessary.

Grade 1-10

Day 35: Rest, Cheat Day—Eat whatever you want, in moderation. Remember meal frequency!

Total Score for the Week

Remember, your score for the week should be at least 48! If your effort has been good, you'll see the difference in your body.

Week 6

The final week for endurance training. Next week you will begin power strength training.

Day 36: Endurance training. Continue to build muscle and get the heart rate moving. Also, perform thirty minutes of cardiovascular training.

EAT: Lean protein, slow-releasing carbohydrate, and vegetable every three to three and a half hours. Drink a minimum of sixty-four ounces of water and take a fiber supplement. Drink a meal replacement shake if necessary.

Grade 1-10

Day 37: Twenty minutes of cardiovascular training on your own. Make sure that you are moving at a moderate pace.

EAT: Protein Day. Lean protein and a vegetable every three to three and a half hours. Consume a minimum of sixty-four ounces of water and take a fiber supplement. To accelerate fat loss, don't eat carbohydrates on non-weight training days. Eat a larger portion of lean protein and vegetables. Drink a meal replacement shake if necessary.

Grade 1-10

Day 38: Endurance training. Continue to build muscle and get the heart rate moving. Also, perform thirty minutes of cardiovascular training.

EAT: Lean protein, slow-releasing carbohydrate, and vegetable every three to three and a half hours. Drink a minimum of sixty-four ounces of water and take a fiber supplement. Drink a meal replacement shake if necessary.

Grade 1-10

Day 39: Twenty minutes of cardiovascular training on your own. Make sure that you are moving at a moderate pace.

EAT: Protein Day. Lean protein and a vegetable every three to three and a half hours. Consume a minimum of sixty-four ounces of water and take a fiber supplement. Drink a meal replacement shake if necessary.

Grade 1-10

Day 40: Endurance training. Continue to build muscle and get the heart rate moving. Also, perform thirty minutes of cardiovascular training.

EAT: Lean protein, slow-releasing carbohydrate, and vegetable every three to three and a half hours. Drink a minimum of sixty-four ounces of water and take a fiber supplement. Drink a meal replacement shake if necessary.

Grade 1-10

Day 41: Twenty minutes of cardiovascular training on your own. Make sure that you are moving at a moderate pace.

EAT: Protein Day. Lean protein and a vegetable every three to three and a half hours. Consume a minimum of sixty-four ounces of water and take a fiber supplement. Drink a meal replacement shake if necessary.

Grade 1-10 []

Day 42: Rest, Cheat Day—Eat whatever you want, in moderation. Remember meal frequency!

Total Score for the Week []

Congratulations! You've made it through the second segment. Give yourself a pat on the back, and keep up the good work!

Week 7

Power strength training. Remember, the more muscle you have, the more your metabolism will increase. For the next three weeks you're going to cut back on cardiovascular training because of the increased demand of strength training.

Day 43: Power strength training. Focusing on muscle growth to increase your metabolism. Perform twenty minutes of cardiovascular training.

EAT: Lean protein, slow-releasing carbohydrate, and vegetable every three to three and a half hours. Drink a minimum of sixty-four ounces of water and take a fiber supplement. Drink a meal replacement shake if necessary.

Grade 1-10 []

Day 44: Fifteen minutes of cardiovascular training on your own. Make sure that you are moving at a moderate pace.

EAT: Protein Day. Lean protein and a vegetable every three to three and a half hours. Consume a minimum of sixty-four ounces of water and take a fiber supplement. To accelerate fat loss, don't eat carbohydrates on non-weight training days. Eat a larger portion of lean protein and vegetables. Drink a meal replacement shake if necessary.

Grade 1-10 ☐

Day 45: Power strength training. Focusing on muscle growth to increase your metabolism. Perform twenty minutes of cardiovascular training.

EAT: Lean protein, slow-releasing carbohydrate, and vegetable every three to three and a half hours. Drink a minimum of sixty-four ounces of water and take a fiber supplement. Drink a meal replacement shake if necessary.

Grade 1-10 ☐

Day 46: Fifteen minutes of cardiovascular training on your own. Make sure that you are moving at a moderate pace.

EAT: Protein Day. Lean protein and a vegetable every three to three and a half hours. Consume a minimum of sixty-four ounces of water and take a fiber supplement. Drink a meal replacement shake if necessary.

Grade 1-10 ☐

Day 47: Power strength training. Focusing on muscle growth to increase your metabolism. Perform twenty minutes of cardiovascular training.

EAT: Lean protein, slow-releasing carbohydrate, and vegetable every three to three and a half hours. Drink a minimum of sixty-four ounces of water and take a fiber supplement. Drink a meal replacement shake if necessary.

Grade 1-10 ☐

Day 48: Fifteen minutes of cardiovascular training on your own. Make sure that you are moving at a moderate pace.

EAT: Protein Day. Lean protein and a vegetable every three to three and a half hours. Consume a minimum of sixty-four ounces of water and take a fiber supplement. Drink a meal replacement shake if necessary.

Grade 1-10 ☐

Day 49: Rest, Cheat Day—Eat whatever you want, in moderation. Remember meal frequency!

Total Score for the Week ☐

How do you like power strength training? Your body is continuing to shape, tone and lose fat.

Week 8

Power strength training. For the next two weeks you will continue to cut back on cardiovascular training because of the increased demand of strength training.

Day 50: Power strength training. Focusing on muscle growth to increase your metabolism. Perform twenty minutes of cardiovascular training.

EAT: Lean protein, slow-releasing carbohydrate, and vegetable every three to three and a half hours. Consume a minimum of sixty-four ounces of water and take a fiber supplement. Drink a meal replacement shake if necessary.

Grade 1-10 ☐

Day 51: Fifteen minutes of cardiovascular training on your own. Make sure that you are moving at a moderate pace.

EAT: Protein Day. Lean protein and a vegetable every three to three and a half hours. Consume a minimum of sixty-four ounces of water and take a fiber supplement. To accelerate fat loss, do not eat carbohydrates on non-weight training days. Eat a larger portion of lean protein and vegetables. Drink a meal replacement shake if necessary.

Grade 1-10 ☐

Day 52: Power strength training. Focusing on muscle growth to increase your metabolism. Perform twenty minutes of cardiovascular training.

EAT: Lean protein, slow-releasing carbohydrate, and vegetable every three to three and a half hours. Drink a minimum of sixty-four ounces of water and take a fiber supplement. Drink a meal replacement shake if necessary.

Grade 1-10

Day 53: Fifteen minutes of cardiovascular training on your own. Make sure that you are moving at a moderate pace.

EAT: Protein Day. Lean protein and a vegetable every three to three and a half hours. Consume a minimum of sixty-four ounces of water and take a fiber supplement. Drink a meal replacement shake if necessary.

Grade 1-10

Day 54: Power strength training. Focusing on muscle growth to increase your metabolism. Perform twenty minutes of cardiovascular training.

EAT: Lean protein, slow-releasing carbohydrate, and vegetable every three to three and a half hours. Drink a minimum of sixty-four ounces of water and take a fiber supplement. Drink a meal replacement shake if necessary.

Grade 1-10

Day 55: Fifteen minutes of cardiovascular training on your own. Make sure that you are moving at a moderate pace.

EAT: Protein Day. Lean protein and a vegetable every three to three and a half hours. Consume a minimum of sixty-four ounces of water and take a fiber supplement. Drink a meal replacement shake if necessary.

Grade 1-10

Day 56: Rest, Cheat Day—Eat whatever you want, in moderation. Remember meal frequency!

Total Score for the Week [   ]

Keep gaining strength! One more week of power strength training and we will shift back to circuit training.

Week 9

This is the last week of power strength training. You will continue to build the important lean muscle tissue.

Day 57: Power strength training. Focusing on muscle growth to increase your metabolism. Perform twenty minutes of cardiovascular training.

EAT: Lean protein, slow-releasing carbohydrate, and vegetable every three to three and a half hours. Drink a minimum of sixty-four ounces of water and take a fiber supplement. Drink a meal replacement shake if necessary.

Grade 1-10 [   ]

Day 58: Fifteen minutes of cardiovascular training on your own. Make sure that you are moving at a moderate pace.

EAT: Protein day. Lean protein and a vegetable every three to three and a half hours. Drink a minimum of sixty-four ounces of water and take a fiber supplement. To accelerate fat loss, don't eat carbohydrates on non-weight training days. Eat a larger portion of lean protein and vegetables. Drink a meal replacement shake if necessary.

Grade 1-10 [   ]

Day 59: Power strength training. Focusing on muscle growth to increase your metabolism. Perform twenty minutes of cardiovascular training.

EAT: Lean protein, slow-releasing carbohydrate, and vegetable every three to three and a half hours. Drink a minimum of sixty-four

ounces of water and take a fiber supplement. Drink a meal replacement shake if necessary.

Grade 1-10 ☐

Day 60: Fifteen minutes of cardiovascular training on your own. Make sure that you are moving at a moderate pace.

EAT: Protein day. Lean protein and a vegetable every three to three and a half hours. Drink a minimum of sixty-four ounces of water and take a fiber supplement. Drink a meal replacement shake if necessary.

Grade 1-10 ☐

Day 61: Power strength training. Focusing on muscle growth to increase your metabolism. Perform twenty minutes of cardiovascular training.

EAT: Lean protein, slow-releasing carbohydrate, and vegetable every three to three and a half hours. Drink a minimum of sixty-four ounces of water and take a fiber supplement. Drink a meal replacement shake if necessary.

Grade 1-10 ☐

Day 62: Fifteen minutes of cardiovascular training on your own. Make sure that you are moving at a moderate pace.

EAT: Protein day. Lean protein and a vegetable every three to three and a half hours. Drink a minimum of sixty-four ounces of water and take a fiber supplement. Drink a meal replacement shake if necessary.

Grade 1-10 ☐

Day 63: Rest, Cheat Day—Eat whatever you want, in moderation. Remember meal frequency!

Total Score for the Week ☐

Congratulations! You've made it through the first phase of the system. Now your metabolism should be burning fuel quickly. In the second phase, body fat is going to decrease at a faster pace. Keep up the good work!

Week 10

Remember, if your workouts get off schedule from what is on the "game plan," just make sure that you are weight training three times per week and cardiovascular training six times per week. In order to promote nutritional caloric variation, you are going to eliminate protein day for the next three weeks.

Day 64: Circuit training: designed to build lean muscle tissue and increase the metabolism. Perform twenty-five minutes of cardiovascular training.

EAT: Lean protein, slow-releasing carbohydrate, and vegetable every three to three and a half hours. Drink a minimum of sixty-four ounces of water and take a fiber supplement. Drink a meal replacement shake if necessary.

Grade 1-10

Day 65: Twenty minutes of cardiovascular training on your own. Make sure that you are moving at a moderate pace

EAT: Lean protein, slow-releasing carbohydrate, and vegetable every three to three and a half hours. Drink a minimum of sixty-four ounces of water and take a fiber supplement. Drink a meal replacement shake if necessary.

Grade 1-10

Day 66: Perform circuit training and twenty-five minutes of cardiovascular training.

EAT: Lean protein, slow-releasing carbohydrate, and vegetable every three to three and a half hours. Drink a minimum of sixty-four ounces of water and take a fiber supplement. Drink a meal replacement shake if necessary.

Grade 1-10

Day 67: Twenty minutes of cardiovascular training on your own. Make sure that you are moving at a moderate pace.

EAT: Lean protein, slow-releasing carbohydrate, and vegetable every three to three and a half hours. Drink a minimum of sixty-four ounces of water and take a fiber supplement. Drink a meal replacement shake if necessary.

Grade 1-10

Day 68: Perform circuit training and twenty-five minutes of cardiovascular training.

EAT: Lean protein, slow-releasing carbohydrate, and vegetable every three to three and a half hours. Drink a minimum of sixty-four ounces of water and take a fiber supplement. Drink a meal replacement shake if necessary.

Grade 1-10

Day 69: Twenty minutes of cardiovascular training on your own. Make sure that you are moving at a moderate pace.

EAT: Lean protein, slow-releasing carbohydrate, and vegetable every three to three and a half hours. Drink a minimum of sixty-four ounces of water and take a fiber supplement. Drink a meal replacement shake if necessary.

Grade 1-10

Day 70: Rest, Cheat Day—Eat whatever you want, in moderation. Remember meal frequency!

Total Score for the Week

Your total score for the week should not be less than 48.

Week 11

Your body should be conditioned to working out and eating supportively. If you're having trouble, please take the time to reread the book or consult with your trainer.

Day 71: Circuit training: designed to build lean muscle tissue and increase metabolism. Perform twenty-five minutes of cardiovascular training.

EAT: Lean protein, slow-releasing carbohydrate, and vegetable every three to three and a half hours. Drink a minimum of sixty-four ounces of water and take a fiber supplement. Drink a meal replacement shake if necessary.

Grade 1-10

Day 72: Twenty minutes of cardiovascular training on your own. Make sure that you are moving at a moderate pace.

EAT: Lean protein, slow-releasing carbohydrate, and vegetable every three to three and a half hours. Drink a minimum of sixty-four ounces of water and take a fiber supplement. Drink a meal replacement shake if necessary.

Grade 1-10

Day 73: Circuit training: designed to build lean muscle tissue and increase metabolism. Perform twenty-five minutes of cardiovascular training.

EAT: Lean protein, slow-releasing carbohydrate, and vegetable every three to three and a half hours. Drink a minimum of sixty-four ounces of water and take a fiber supplement. Drink a meal replacement shake if necessary.

Grade 1-10

Day 74: Twenty minutes of cardiovascular training on your own. Make sure that you are moving at a moderate pace.

EAT: Lean protein, slow-releasing carbohydrate, and vegetable every three to three and a half hours. Drink a minimum of sixty-four ounces of water and take a fiber supplement. Drink a meal replacement shake if necessary.

Grade 1-10

Day 75: Circuit training: designed to build lean muscle tissue and increase metabolism. Perform twenty-five minutes of cardiovascular training.

EAT: Lean protein, slow-releasing carbohydrate, and vegetable every three to three and a half hours. Drink a minimum of sixty-four ounces of water and take a fiber supplement. Drink a meal replacement shake if necessary.

Grade 1-10

Day 76: Twenty minutes of cardiovascular training on your own. Make sure that you are moving at a moderate pace.

EAT: Lean protein, slow-releasing carbohydrate, and vegetable every three to three and a half hours. Drink a minimum of sixty-four ounces of water and take a fiber supplement. Drink a meal replacement shake if necessary.

Grade 1-10

Day 77: Rest, Cheat Day—Eat whatever you want, in moderation. Remember meal frequency!

Total Score for the Week

Your clothes should fit dramatically different. You're improving your body and the quality of your life!

Week 12

This is the last week of circuit training in this phase. Finish strong!

Day 78: Circuit training: designed to build lean muscle tissue and increase metabolism. Perform twenty-five minutes of cardiovascular training.

EAT: Lean protein, slow-releasing carbohydrate, and vegetable every three to three and a half hours. Drink a minimum of sixty-four ounces of water and take a fiber supplement. Drink a meal replacement shake if necessary.

Grade 1-10

Day 79: Twenty minutes of cardiovascular training on your own. Make sure that you are moving at a moderate pace.

EAT: Lean protein, slow-releasing carbohydrate, and vegetable every three to three and a half hours. Drink a minimum of sixty-four ounces of water and take a fiber supplement. Drink a meal replacement shake if necessary.

Grade 1-10   ☐

Day 80: Circuit training: designed to build lean muscle tissue and increase metabolism. Perform twenty-five minutes of cardiovascular training.

EAT: Lean protein, slow-releasing carbohydrate, and vegetable every three to three and a half hours. Drink a minimum of sixty-four ounces of water and take a fiber supplement. Drink a meal replacement shake if necessary.

Grade 1-10   ☐

Day 81: Twenty minutes of cardiovascular training on your own. Make sure that you are moving at a moderate pace.

EAT: Lean protein, slow-releasing carbohydrate, and vegetable every three to three and a half hours. Drink a minimum of sixty-four ounces of water and take a fiber supplement. Drink a meal replacement shake if necessary.

Grade 1-10   ☐

Day 82: Circuit training: designed to build lean muscle tissue and increase metabolism. Perform twenty-five minutes of cardiovascular training.

EAT: Lean protein, slow-releasing carbohydrate, and vegetable every three to three and a half hours. Drink a minimum of sixty-four ounces of water and take a fiber supplement. Drink a meal replacement shake if necessary.

Grade 1-10   ☐

Day 83: Twenty minutes of cardiovascular training on your own. Make sure that you are moving at a moderate pace.

EAT: Lean protein, slow-releasing carbohydrate, and vegetable every three to three and a half hours. Drink a minimum of sixty-four ounces of water and take a fiber supplement. Drink a meal replacement shake if necessary.

Grade 1-10

Day 84: Rest, Cheat Day—Eat whatever you want, in moderation. Remember meal frequency!

Total Score for the Week

Let's begin to perform endurance training again and really accelerate your results!

Week 13

You will once again perform endurance training with shortened rest periods. New exercises are added and protein day returns for caloric variation to accelerate results.

Day 85: Endurance training. Continue to build muscle and get the heart rate moving! Perform thirty minutes of cardiovascular training.

EAT: Lean protein, slow-releasing carbohydrate, and vegetable every three to three and a half hours. Drink a minimum of sixty-four ounces of water and take a fiber supplement. Drink a meal replacement shake if necessary.

Grade 1-10

Day 86: Twenty minutes of cardiovascular training on your own. Make sure that you are moving at a moderate pace.

EAT: Protein day. Lean protein and a vegetable every three to three and a half hours. Consume a minimum of sixty-four ounces of water and take a fiber supplement. To accelerate fat loss, don't eat carbohydrates on non-weight training days. Eat a larger portion of lean protein and vegetables. Drink a meal replacement shake if necessary.

Grade 1-10

Day 87: Perform endurance training and thirty minutes of cardiovascular training.

EAT: Lean protein, slow-releasing carbohydrate, and vegetable every three to three and a half hours. Drink a minimum of sixty-four ounces of water and take a fiber supplement. Drink a meal replacement shake if necessary.

Grade 1-10

Day 88: Twenty minutes of cardiovascular training on your own. Make sure that you are moving at a moderate pace.

EAT: Protein day. Lean protein and a vegetable every three to three and a half hours. Consume a minimum of sixty-four ounces of water and take a fiber supplement. Drink a meal replacement shake if necessary.

Grade 1-10

Day 89: Perform endurance training and thirty minutes of cardiovascular training.

EAT: Lean protein, slow-releasing carbohydrate, and vegetable every three to three and a half hours. Drink a minimum of sixty-four ounces of water and take a fiber supplement. Drink a meal replacement shake if necessary.

Grade 1-10

Day 90: Twenty minutes of cardiovascular training on your own. Make sure that you are moving at a moderate pace.

EAT: Protein day. Lean protein and a vegetable every three to three and a half hours. Consume a minimum of sixty-four ounces of water and take a fiber supplement. Drink a meal replacement shake if necessary.

Grade 1-10

Day 91: Rest, Cheat Day—Eat whatever you want, in moderation. Remember meal frequency!

Total Score for the Week

You should begin to notice a big change in your appearance!

Week 14

You will once again perform endurance training with shortened rest periods. Make sure that you're keeping an accurate and honest evaluation of your efforts!

Day 92: Endurance training. Continue to build muscle and get the heart rate moving! Perform thirty minutes of cardiovascular training.

EAT: Lean protein, slow-releasing carbohydrate, and vegetable every three to three and a half hours. Drink a minimum of sixty-four ounces of water and take a fiber supplement. Drink a meal replacement shake if necessary.

Grade 1-10

Day 93: Twenty minutes of cardiovascular training on your own. Make sure that you are moving at a moderate pace.

EAT: Protein day. Lean protein and a vegetable every three to three and a half hours. Consume a minimum of sixty-four ounces of water and take a fiber supplement. To accelerate fat loss, don't eat carbohydrates on non-weight training days. Eat a larger portion of lean protein and vegetables. Drink a meal replacement shake if necessary.

Grade 1-10

Day 94: Endurance training. Continue to build muscle and get the heart rate moving. Perform thirty minutes of cardiovascular training.

EAT: Lean protein, slow-releasing carbohydrate, and vegetable every three to three and a half hours. Drink a minimum of sixty-four

ounces of water and take a fiber supplement. Drink a meal replacement shake if necessary.

Grade 1-10

Day 95: Twenty minutes of cardiovascular training on your own. Make sure that you are moving at a moderate pace.

EAT: Protein day. Lean protein and a vegetable every three to three and a half hours. Consume a minimum of sixty-four ounces of water and take a fiber supplement. Drink a meal replacement shake if necessary.

Grade 1-10

Day 96: Endurance training. Continue to build muscle and get the heart rate moving. Perform thirty minutes of cardiovascular training.

EAT: Lean protein, slow-releasing carbohydrate, and vegetable every three to three and a half hours. Drink a minimum of sixty-four ounces of water and take a fiber supplement. Drink a meal replacement shake if necessary.

Grade 1-10

Day 97: Twenty minutes of cardiovascular training on your own. Make sure that you are moving at a moderate pace.

EAT: Protein day. Lean protein and a vegetable every three to three and a half hours. Consume a minimum of sixty-four ounces of water and take a fiber supplement. Drink a meal replacement shake if necessary.

Grade 1-10

Day 98: Rest, Cheat Day—Eat whatever you want, in moderation. Remember meal frequency!

Total Score for the Week

One more week of endurance training and then you are going back to power strength training!

Week 15

Endurance training is performed for the last time in this phase. Your body should be much tighter and more toned than it was fifteen weeks ago. You've kept your commitment!

Day 99: Endurance training. Continue to build muscle and get the heart rate moving! Perform thirty minutes of cardiovascular training.

EAT: Lean protein, slow-releasing carbohydrate, and vegetable every three to three and a half hours. Drink a minimum of sixty-four ounces of water and take a fiber supplement. Drink a meal replacement shake if necessary.

Grade 1-10

Day 100: Twenty minutes of cardiovascular training on your own. Make sure that you are moving at a moderate pace.

EAT: Protein day. Lean protein and a vegetable every three to three and a half hours. Consume a minimum of sixty-four ounces of water and take a fiber supplement. To accelerate fat loss, don't eat carbohydrates on non-weight training days. Eat a larger portion of lean protein and vegetables. Drink a meal replacement shake if necessary.

Grade 1-10

Day 101: Endurance training. Continue to build muscle and get the heart rate moving! Perform thirty minutes of cardiovascular training.

EAT: Lean protein, slow-releasing carbohydrate, and vegetable every three to three and a half hours. Drink a minimum of sixty-four ounces of water and take a fiber supplement. Drink a meal replacement shake if necessary.

Grade 1-10

Day 102: Twenty minutes of cardiovascular training on your own. Make sure that you are moving at a moderate pace.

EAT: Protein day. Lean protein and a vegetable every three to three and a half hours. Consume a minimum of sixty-four ounces of water and take a fiber supplement. Drink a meal replacement shake if necessary.

Grade 1-10

Day 103: Endurance training. Continue to build muscle and get the heart rate moving! Perform thirty minutes of cardiovascular training.

EAT: Lean protein, slow-releasing carbohydrate, and vegetable every three to three and a half hours. Drink a minimum of sixty-four ounces of water and take a fiber supplement. Drink a meal replacement shake if necessary.

Grade 1-10

Day 104: Twenty minutes of cardiovascular training on your own. Make sure that you are moving at a moderate pace.

EAT: Protein day. Lean protein and a vegetable every three to three and a half hours. Consume a minimum of sixty-four ounces of water and take a fiber supplement. Drink a meal replacement shake if necessary.

Grade 1-10

Day 105: Rest, Cheat Day—Eat whatever you want, in moderation. Remember meal frequency!

Total Score for the Week

Time to power it up again! Three weeks of power strength training are coming up!

Week 16

Power strength training. Remember, the more muscle you have, the faster your metabolism will be. (Relax, you won't look like an Olympic power-lifter!) The next three weeks we are going to cut back on cardiovascular training because of the increased demand of strength training.

Day 106: Power strength training. Focusing on muscle growth to increase your metabolism. Perform twenty minutes of cardiovascular training.

EAT: Lean protein, slow-releasing carbohydrate, and vegetable every three to three and a half hours. Drink a minimum of sixty-four ounces of water and take a fiber supplement. Drink a meal replacement shake if necessary.

Grade 1-10

Day 107: Fifteen minutes of cardiovascular training on your own. Make sure that you are moving at a moderate pace.

EAT: Protein day. Lean protein and a vegetable every three to three and a half hours. Consume a minimum of sixty-four ounces of water and take a fiber supplement. To accelerate fat loss, don't eat carbohydrates on non-weight training days. Eat a larger portion of lean protein and vegetables. Drink a meal replacement shake if necessary.

Grade 1-10

Day 108: Perform power strength training and twenty minutes of cardiovascular training

EAT: Lean protein, slow-releasing carbohydrate, and vegetable every three to three and a half hours. Drink a minimum of sixty-four ounces of water and take a fiber supplement. Drink a meal replacement shake if necessary.

Grade 1-10

Day 109: Fifteen minutes of cardiovascular training on your own. Make sure that you are moving at a moderate pace.

EAT: Protein day. Lean protein and a vegetable every three to three and a half hours. Consume a minimum of sixty-four ounces of water and take a fiber supplement. Drink a meal replacement shake if necessary.

Grade 1-10

Day 110: Perform power strength training and twenty minutes of cardiovascular training.

EAT: Lean protein, slow-releasing carbohydrate, and vegetable every three to three and a half hours. Drink a minimum of sixty-four ounces of water and take a fiber supplement. Drink a meal replacement shake if necessary.

Grade 1-10

Day 111: Fifteen minutes of cardiovascular training on your own. Make sure that you are moving at a moderate pace.

EAT: Protein day. Lean protein and a vegetable every three to three and a half hours. Consume a minimum of sixty-four ounces of water and take a fiber supplement. Drink a meal replacement shake if necessary.

Grade 1-10

Day 112: Rest, Cheat Day—Eat whatever you want, in moderation. Remember meal frequency!

Total Score for the Week

When you increase your lean muscle tissue, you'll increase your metabolism and burn more fat!

Week 17

Continue power strength training. After next week, we're going to change the entire system and begin phase three. You have performed admirably and kept your commitment. I applaud you!

Day 113: Power strength training. Focusing on muscle growth to increase your metabolism. Perform twenty minutes of cardiovascular training.

EAT: Lean protein, slow-releasing carbohydrate, and vegetable every three to three and a half hours. Drink a minimum of sixty-four ounces of water and take a fiber supplement. Drink a meal replacement shake if necessary.

Grade 1-10

Day 114: Fifteen minutes of cardiovascular training on your own. Make sure that you are moving at a moderate pace.

EAT: Protein day. Lean protein and a vegetable every three to three and a half hours. Drink a minimum of sixty-four ounces of water and take a fiber supplement. To accelerate fat loss, don't eat carbohydrates on non-weight training days. Eat a larger portion of lean protein and vegetables. Drink a meal replacement shake if necessary.

Grade 1-10

Day 115: Perform power strength training and twenty minutes of cardiovascular training

EAT: Lean protein, slow-releasing carbohydrate, and vegetable every three to three and a half hours. Drink a minimum of sixty-four ounces of water and take a fiber supplement. Drink a meal replacement shake if necessary.

Grade 1-10

Day 116: Fifteen minutes of cardiovascular training on your own. Make sure that you are moving at a moderate pace.

EAT: Protein day. Lean protein and a vegetable every three to three and a half hours. Consume a minimum of sixty-four ounces of water and take a fiber supplement. Drink a meal replacement shake if necessary.

Grade 1-10

Day 117: Perform power strength training and twenty minutes of cardiovascular training

EAT: Lean protein, slow-releasing carbohydrate, and vegetable every three to three and a half hours. Drink a minimum of sixty-four ounces of water and take a fiber supplement. Drink a meal replacement shake if necessary.

Grade 1-10

Day 118: Fifteen minutes of cardiovascular training on your own. Make sure that you are moving at a moderate pace.

EAT: Protein day. Lean protein and a vegetable every three to three and a half hours. Consume a minimum of sixty-four ounces of water and take a fiber supplement. Drink a meal replacement shake if necessary.

Grade 1-10 ☐

Day 119: Rest, Cheat Day—Eat whatever you want, in moderation. Remember meal frequency!

Total Score for the Week ☐

You've worked hard and followed the system well. You should be looking and feeling great!

Week 18

If you are still with me (and I know that only those who truly want to get into better health and fitness are), you have *transformed* your body. You're a different (healthier) person than eighteen weeks ago! You've done wonderfully. I encourage you to keep up the good work!

Day 120: Power strength training. Focusing on muscle growth to increase your metabolism. Perform twenty minutes of cardiovascular training.

EAT: Lean protein, slow-releasing carbohydrate, and vegetable every three to three and a half hours. Drink a minimum of sixty-four ounces of water and take a fiber supplement. Drink a meal replacement shake if necessary.

Grade 1-10 ☐

Day 121: Fifteen minutes of cardiovascular training on your own. Make sure that you are moving at a moderate pace.

EAT: Protein day. Lean protein and a vegetable every three to three and a half hours. Drink a minimum of sixty-four ounces of water and take a fiber supplement. To accelerate fat loss, don't eat carbohydrates on non-weight training days. Eat a larger portion of lean protein and vegetables. Drink a meal replacement shake if necessary.

Grade 1-10

Day 122: Perform power strength training and twenty minutes of cardiovascular training

EAT: Lean protein, slow-releasing carbohydrate, and vegetable every three to three and a half hours. Drink a minimum of sixty-four ounces of water and take a fiber supplement. Drink a meal replacement shake if necessary.

Grade 1-10

Day 123: Fifteen minutes of cardiovascular training on your own. Make sure that you are moving at a moderate pace.

EAT: Protein day. Lean protein and a vegetable every three to three and a half hours. Drink a minimum of sixty-four ounces of water and take a fiber supplement. Drink a meal replacement shake if necessary.

Grade 1-10

Day 124: Perform power strength training and twenty minutes of cardiovascular training

EAT: Lean protein, slow-releasing carbohydrate, and vegetable every three to three and a half hours. Drink a minimum of sixty-four ounces of water and take a fiber supplement. Drink a meal replacement shake if necessary.

Grade 1-10

Day 125: Fifteen minutes of cardiovascular training on your own. Make sure that you are moving at a moderate pace.

EAT: Protein day. Lean protein and a vegetable every three to three and a half hours. Drink a minimum of sixty-four ounces of water and take a fiber supplement. Drink a meal replacement shake if necessary.

Grade 1-10

Day 126: Rest, Cheat Day—Eat whatever you want, in moderation. Remember meal frequency!

Total Score for the Week

Way to finish strong! Good job! Let's set new goals to achieve!

Chapter XIX

A visual guide to the exercises

Abs

Ball crunch.

2. Pull the shoulders off the floor while keeping the belly button down.

1. Position your legs over the top of the ball and lift.

2. Exhale as you press the belly button into the floor.

_ Sit up

2. Pull the shoulders off the floor while keeping the belly button down.

1. Exhale as you press the belly button into the floor.

Hip extensions- supine

1. Exhale as you fire the legs to the ceiling.

Ball sit up

1. Exhale as you press the belly button into the floor.

2. Sit up while keeping the belly button pressed down.

Vertical knee raise- alt.

2. Exhale as you press the belly button into the bench.

Alternate

1. Start with both knees raised to 90°

3. Raise one leg at a time. Fire the knee high into the chest and hold for 1-2 sec.

Reverse twist

1. Exhale as you press the belly button into the floor.

2. Exhale as you pull the knees across the body to the opposite shoulder.

Ball- Twisting crunch

2. Exhale as you pull the shoulder across the body to the opposite knee. Keep the belly down during the crunch.

1. Exhale as you press the belly button into the floor.

Twisting jack knife

Exhale as you pull both across the body to the opposite shoulder. Keep the back rounded during the crunch.

Ball- Knee rotation

1. Position your legs around the medicine tightly.

2. Slowly rotate the hips from side to side. Increase the range of motion on each repetition.

Ball- Torso twist

Slowly rotate the torso keeping the hips stable. Increase range of motion on each repetition.

Lat pulldown-neutral

-keep back straight
-chest out
-head up

neutral grip

Exhale and squeeze the shoulder blades together as you pull the bar to the sternum. Hold at bottom for 1-2 sec.

Lat pulldown-overhand

pronation grip

Exhale and squeeze the shoulder blades together as you pull the bar to the clavicle. Hold at bottom for 1-2 sec.

One arm row-DB

neutral grip

Exhale and squeeze the back as you pull the dumbbell to the chest. Elbow tight to the body. Hold at top for 1-2 sec.

Pull-up

wide grip
pronation grip

Exhale and squeeze the shoulder blades together as you pull your chest to the bar Hold at chest for 1-2 sec.

Bent over row-DB

pronation

Exhale and squeeze the shoulder blades together as you pull the dumbbells to the nipple line. Hold at chest for 1-2 sec.

Deadlift-BB

-keep back straight
-chest out
-head up

Exhale and slowly lift the bar from the floor while maintaining a lower back arch.

157

Upper back

Seated rope row to neck

on pulley
with cable

-keep back
straight
-chest out
-head up

Exhale and squeeze the shoulder blades together as you pull the rope to the clavicle. Hold at top for 1-2 sec.

Upright row

-keep back
straight
-chest out
-head up

Exhale and squeeze the shoulder blades together as you pull the bar to the chin. Hold at top for 1-2 sec.

1st Pull

-keep back
straight
-chest out
-head up

Explosive upward motion. Exhale and squeeze the shoulder blades together as you thrust the bar to the chin. Lower the bar under control.

Lower back

Superman

Exhale and raise the arms and leg simultaneously from the lower back. Hold at top for 1-2 sec.

Jimmy Olsen

Exhale and raise the torso from the lower back. Keep the hips pressed down. Hold at top for 1-2 sec.

Good Morning -BB

1. Position the bar between the shoulders and the neck. Knees at 15˚ bend.

2. Push the buttocks straight back as you start your decent. DO NOT BEND KNEES.

-keep back
straight
-chest out
-head up

3. Arch your lower back and lower the torso to 90˚.

Legs

Split Squat -BB

1. Position the bar between the shoulders and the neck.

2. Split your legs 3-4 feet apart.

*When properly done you will feel a stretch in the rear hip flexor.

2. Arch your lower back and push the elbows forward as you lower to 90˚.

Lunge -BB

1. Position the bar between the shoulders and the neck.

2. Step forward heel to toe as you start your decent.

3. Arch your lower back and push the chest out as you lower to 90˚.

Ball squat

1. Position the ball in the small of back.

2. Push the knees forward over the toes as you start your decent.

90°

3. Arch your lower back and push the buttocks toward the wall as you lower to 90˚.

Squat -BB

1. Position the bar between the shoulders and the neck.

2. Push the knees forward over the toes as you start your decent.

Full squat

3. Arch your lower back and lower the buttocks to 90˚.

Legs, continued

Hack squat-BB

2. Push the knees forward over the toes as you start your decent.

1. Position the bar under the buttocks. "You may want to put a 2"x4" under your heels for balance.

3. Arch your lower back and push the buttocks backwards as you lower to 90˚.

Ball- split squat

1. Position the rear leg on the ball.

2. Split your front leg 4+ feet apart.

"When properly done you will feel a stretch in the rear hip flexor.

2. Push your front foot forward and arch your lower back as you lower your body.

Lateral squat-BB

2. Push the knees side to side outside the toes as you begin.

1. Position the bar between the shoulders and the neck. Feet turned out slightly.

3. Keep the elbows even and pushed forward during the motion.

Lunge -BB

Walk backward

1. Step backward toe to heel as you start your walk.

2. Arch your lower back and push the chest out as you lower to 90˚.

3. Step the front leg back to return to the original position.

Side step up-BB

2. Push the "up" knee forward over the toes as you start your accent. Side

1. Position the "up" foot on the bench. The "down" foot on the floor TO THE SIDE OF THE BENCH.-with the toes curled up.

3. Arch your lower back and keep the head up as you step up on to the bench. Lower slowly.

Front step up-DB

2. Push the knees forward over the toes as you start your accent.

one foot on the bench

front step-up

1. Position the "up" foot on the bench. The "down" foot on the floor- with the toes curled up.

3. Arch your lower back and keep the head up as you step up on to the bench. Lower slowly.

Hamstrings

 Calves

Toe raise-machine

1. Position the bar between the shoulders and the neck. Lock the knees. Ball of the foot on the 2"x4".

2. Raise the body with the toes as high as possible.

3. Lower the body until the heels are stretched fully.

Leg curl

Place Achilles' tendon under rear pad, knee to the rear of middle pad.

Exhale and squeeze as you curl the weight to the buttocks. Lower slowly for 2 seconds.

Ball- low back bridge

Place feet flat on top of the medicine ball.

Exhale and squeeze the buttocks as you raise your hips. Hold at the top for 2 seconds.

Chest

Bench Press-DB

1. Position the shoulder blades on the bench. Dumbbells on the chest. Elbows at 90° Feet flat on floor at all times.

2. Exhale and press the dumbbells from the chest to a locked elbow position. Move slowly in a straight controlled manner.

Bench Press-BB

1. Position the grip 14" apart. Wrist straight and locked. Feet flat on floor at all times.

2. Exhale and press the dumbbells from the collar bone to a locked elbow position. Move slowly in a straight controlled manner.

Parallel bar dip

1. Start with the body off the floor. Elbows bent. Chest and head up. Knees bent and behind the torso.

thumb inside

2. Exhale and thrust the body to a locked elbow position. Pause 1 sec. Lower slowly in a straight controlled manner.

Ball bench press-DB

1. Position the shoulder blades on the ball. Dumbbells on the chest. Elbows at 90° Feet flat on floor at all times.

2. Exhale and press the dumbbells from the chest to a locked elbow position. Move slowly in a straight controlled manner.

Decline push up- loaded

1. Start with the body off the floor. Hands 14" apart. Elbows locked and straight. Chest and head up. Weight on mid back. Feet on bench.

2. Inhale and lower the body to the floor. Pause momentarily. Feel the chest stretch.

3. Exhale and press the body to the start position.

Flye-DB

1. Start with the dumbbells over your chest —elbows locked. Palms parallel. Feet flat on floor at all times.

2. Inhale and lower the dumbbells to a locked 60° open elbow position. Move slowly and feel the chest stretch.

3. Exhale and raise the dumbbells to the start position. Move slowly in an arched, controlled manner.

Upper chest

1. Start with the dumbbells over your chest —elbows locked. Feet flat on floor at all times.

Incline flye-DB

3. Exhale and raise the dumbbells to the start position. Move slowly in an arched, controlled manner.

2. Inhale and lower the dumbbells to a locked 60° open elbow position. Move slowly and feel the chest stretch.

1. Start with the dumbbells over your chest —elbows locked. Palms facing down. Feet flat on floor at all times.

Incline flye-DB

incline fly

3. Exhale and raise the dumbbells to the start position. Move slowly in an arched, controlled manner.

2. Inhale and lower the dumbbells to a locked 60° open elbow position. Move slowly and feel the chest stretch.

Ball shoulder press-DB

1. Start seated on the ball, back arched chest out. Dumbbells on the shoulders. Elbows at 90° Feet flat on floor at all times.

2. Exhale and press the dumbbells to a locked elbow position. Move slowly in a straight controlled manner.

Push press-BB

push on knees

Explosive upward motion. Begin with bent knees. Exhale and press the bar from the collar bone to an elbow locked position. Lower the bar slowly under control.

Reverse flye-DB

-keep back straight
-chest out
-head up

Exhale and squeeze the shoulder blades together as you arch the dumbbells from the center to the side. Hold at the top for 1-2 sec. Lower slowly.

Ball shoulder press-DB

1. Start seated on a chair or bench. Dumbbells on the shoulders. Elbows at 90° Feet flat on floor at all times.

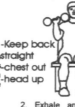

-Keep back straight
chest out
head up

2. Exhale and press the dumbbells from the shoulders to a locked elbow position. Move slowly in a straight controlled manner.

Rotators

Seated external rotation-DB

Exhale as you rotate the dumbbell from the thigh to the side. Keep the elbow fixed at 90° Rotate 3 seconds up and down.

Cuban Press-BB

1. Start with a barbell at waist level. Upright row the bar to the nipple line.

2. Press the bar over the head in a rotational motion, locking the elbows at the top. Reverse these steps as you lower the bar.

Standing side raise-DB

Exhale as you arch the dumbbell from the thigh to the side. Keep the elbow locked. Hold at the top for 1-2 sec. Lower slowly.

Lying internal rotation-DB

Exhale as you rotate the dumbbell from the face level to a point perpendicular to the body. Keep the elbow fixed at 90° Rotate 3 seconds up and down.

165

Standing hammer grip curls-DB -

1. Start with dumbbells at waist level, thumbs up. Slowly curl the dumbbells to the nipple line while keeping your elbows fixated at your sides

2. Hold for 2 seconds then lower the dumbbells slowly to a full elbow lockout at the bottom.

Standing curls- EZ bar

1. Start with a barbell at waist level. Curl the bar to the nipple line.

2. Hold for 2 seconds then lower the bar slowly to a full elbow lockout at the bottom.

Seated curls-EZ bar

1. Start with a close grip on the curl bar. Elbows at 45°. Inhale and lower the bar to the elbow straight position 180°.

2. Exhale as you return the bar slowly back to the top position.

Alternating curls- DB

1. Start with a dumbbell at bottom and one at the top.

2. Alternate your motion. Bring one arm down as the other arm goes up. Exhale as the weight goes up.

Lying extension-DB (skull crusher)

1. Position the shoulder blades on the bench. Dumbbells on the bench next to the ears. Elbows pointed to the ceiling. Feet flat on floor at all times.

neutral grip

2. Exhale and press the dumbbells from the bench to a locked elbow position. Move slowly in a straight controlled manner.

Ball lying extension-DB (skull crusher)

1. Position the shoulder blades on the ball. Close grip, EZ bar begins at the forehead. Elbows pointed to the ceiling. Feet flat on floor at all times.

2. Exhale and press the bar from the forehead to a locked elbow position. Move slowly in a straight controlled manner.

Bench dip, feet elevated, pronated

1. Start with the arms shoulder width behind the torso. Elbows bent. 90˚. Chest and head up. Knees locked and heels on the box or bench.

2. Exhale and thrust the body to a locked elbow position. Pause 1 sec. then inhale and lower slowly in a straight controlled manner.

Bench dip, feet on ball, semi supinated

1. Start with the arms shoulder width behind the torso. Elbows bent. 90˚. Chest and head up. Knees lbent and feet flat on the medicne ball.

2. Exhale and thrust the body to a locked elbow position. Pause 1 sec. then inhale and lower slowly in a straight controlled manner.

Seated extension-DB

1. Start seated on a chair or bench. Elbows bent & stretched to lowest position with dumbell. Feet flat on floor at all times.

2. Exhale and press the dumbbell to a locked elbow position. Pause. Inhale & lower the DB slowly to the starting position.

Cable pushdown

1. Start standing with your shoulders back, knees slightly bent, feet shoulder width and elbows bent at 30˚. 6" wide grip.

semi-pronation

2. Exhale and press the bar to a locked elbow position. Pause. Inhale & raise the bar slowly to the starting position.

167

Flexibility

Hamstrings

1. Lie on back. Then lift active leg toward your head. (watch that the knee is bent at all times) Deepen the stretch to a level 7 intensity and hold for 30 seconds.

2. Resist isometrically as you exhale and push your leg forward against your hold. Push for 10 seconds starting at 50% and build up to 100%. Keep your hips flat as you push.

3. Repeat 2-3 more times.

hold top
leg down

Shoulder clock

1. Lie on one hip. Rotate the top leg over the bottom. HOLD DOWN WITH BOTTOM ARM.

2. Start the motion with both hands together at the three OR nine o'clock positions. Glide top hand around the clock to the other side. Flip hand at 12 o'clock.

3. Repeat 20 times.

Lower back

1. Sit, legs extended knees slightly bent. With lower back straight, roll the ball slowly from side to side.

Standing shoulder clock

1. Stand with heels, buttocks, shoulders and head against wall.

2. Start the motion with both hands at the six o'clock position and simultaneously glide hand around the clock to 12 o'clock. Flip hands around 3 and 9 respectively.

3. Repeat 20 times.

Quadriceps (thigh)

1. Bend and lift active leg toward your buttocks. Deepen the stretch in the thigh to a level 7 intensity and hold for 30 seconds.

2. Resist isometrically, as you exhale and straighten your leg against your hold. Push for 10 seconds starting at 50% and build up to 100%. Keep your hips straight as you push.

3. Repeat 2-3 more times.

Shoulder capsule stretch

1. Kneel on 1 leg in front of a table. Arms behind body at roughly shoulder height-hands flat. Lean down and away to deepen stretch. Squeeze shoulder blades together while stretching.

2. Hold 20 seconds.

Standing chest stretch

1. Stand in corner with elbows at 90°. Lean into corner to deepen stretch. Squeeze shoulder blades together while stretching.

2. Hold 20 seconds.

Psoas (hip flexor)

1. Bend and lift active leg – position on step or block. Bend the forward knee over the forward toe-keep feet flat. Lean forward and deepen the stretch in the REAR HIP to a level 7 intensity and hold for 30 seconds.

2. Resist isometrically, as you exhale and straighten your leg against your hold. Push for 10 seconds starting at 50% and build up to 100%. Keep your hips straight as you push.

3. Repeat 2-3 more times.

Triceps (back of upper arm)

1. Use towel, rubber band or rope. Pull top hand downward behind neck. Deepen the stretch in the tricep to a level 7 intensity and hold for 30 seconds. KEEPING THE SAME POSITION pull the towel toward the ceiling to raise the bottom hand to the sky – deepin to a leval 7 and hold.

2. Resist isometrically, as you exhale and straighten your leg against your hold. Push for 10 seconds starting at 50% and build up to 100%. Keep your hips straight as you push.

3. Repeat 2-3 more times.

Gluteus maximus (buttocks)

1. Bend and lift active leg toward your head. Deepen the stretch in the buttocks to a level 7 intensity and hold for 30 seconds.

2. Resist isometrically, as you exhale and straighten your leg against your hold. Push for 10 seconds starting at 50% and build up to 100%. Keep your hips straight as you push.

3. Repeat 2-3 more times.

Quadratus lumborum

1. Bend right knee and place foot flat. Position left ankle on top of right knee. Push right knee toward floor. Deepen the stretch in the hips and back to a level 7 intensity and hold for 30 seconds.

2. Resist isometrically, as you exhale and straighten your leg against your hold. Push for 10 seconds starting at 50% and build up to 100%. Keep your hips straight as you push.

3. Repeat 2-3 more times.

Chapter XX

Chart your progress

Use these workouts as a guideline. Don't get frustrated if some of these exercises are not available to you, just follow along as best as possible. Remember, for assistance, go to our website www.AlessiFit.com. Always begin with weights you can handle. If a weight is too light, you can always add more. If you have any questions, check with a personal trainer.

Good luck and don't ever give up!

Week 1- Circuit Training: **Get the metabolism moving:**
Goal: 3-weeks of Muscle shaping & toning employing a base from which to work. Begin to build Lean Muscle Tissue. Combining big muscles

Exercises

	1	2	3	4	5	6
	lb.X15-20reps	lb.X15-20reps	lb.X15-20reps	lb.X15-20reps	lb.X15-20reps	lb.X15-20reps

Chest/Back/Legs — Warmups: Hamstrings, Thigh, Glute & hip

Workout #1

Set 1						
Set 2						
Set 3						

15 min. cardiovascular exercise at level 5 exertion

Exercises

	1	2	3	4	5	6
	lb.X15-20reps	lb.X15-20reps	lb.X15-20reps	lb.X15-20reps	lb.X15-20reps	lb.X15-20reps

Shoulders/Biceps/Triceps — Warmups: Hamstrings, Thigh, Glute & hip

Workout #2

Set 1						
Set 2						
Set 3						

15 min. cardiovascular exercise at level 5 exertion

Exercises

	1	2	3	4	5	6
	lb.X15-20reps	lb.X15-20reps	lb.X15-20reps	lb.X15-20reps	lb.X15-20reps	lb.X15-20reps

Chest/Back/Legs — Warmups: Hamstrings, Thigh, Glute & hip

Workout #3

Set 1						
Set 2						
Set 3						

Notes:

Week 2: Get the metabolism moving: Circuit Training
Goal: Continue to build LMT to help speed up metabolism.

15 min. cardiovascular exercise at level 5 exertion

20 min. cardiovascular exercise at level 5 exertion

20 min. cardiovascular exercise at level 5 exertion

20 min. cardiovascular exercise at level 5 exertion

Notes:

Week 3

Notes:

Week 4- Endurance Training-Now the body is beginning to b

Goal - 3 Weeks of endurance training with shortened rest periods. This will ensure that the metabolism speeds up.

25 min. cardiovascular exercise at level 5 exertion

Warmups

Chest/Back/Abs

	Assisted low back	Hip flexor	Shoulders	1	2	3	4	5	6
						30sec.fast			Jump rope 30sec.fast
				lb.X12-15reps	lb.X12-15reps	lb.X12-15reps	lb.X12-15reps	lb.X12-15reps	lb.X12-15reps

Workout#10

Set 1	
Set 2	
Set 3	

Exercises

30 min. cardiovascular exercise at level 5 exertion

Warmups

Legs

	Shoulder circles	Hip flexor	Shoulders	1	2	3	4	5	6
	hold top leg down					30sec.fast			Jump rope 30sec.fast
				lb.X12-15reps	lb.X12-15reps	lb.X12-15reps	lb.X12-15reps	lb.X12-15reps	lb.X12-15reps

Workout#11

Set 1	
Set 2	
Set 3	

Exercises

30 min. cardiovascular exercise at level 5 exertion

Warmups

Shoulders/Arms

	Triceps & shoulder static stretch	Hip flexor	Shoulders	1	2	3	4	5	6
						30sec.fast			Jump rope 30sec.fast
				lb.X12-15reps	lb.X12-15reps	lb.X12-15reps	lb.X12-15reps	lb.X12-15reps	lb.X12-15reps

Workout#12

Set 1	
Set 2	
Set 3	

30 min. cardiovascular exercise at level 5 exertion

Notes:

175

Notes:

Week 6

One more week of lactic acid endurance training and then into the POWER Strength Training.

Notes:

Week 7-Power Strength Training

Goal: 3 weeks of strength training focusing on muscle growth. Remember, the more muscle you have, the more fat you will burn.

Women, don't be worried. You will not look like Zena, the muscle chick!

Notes:

Week 8

Goal: 2nd week of strength training focusing on muscle growth. Remember, the more muscle you have, the more fat you will burn.

Notes

Week 9

Torso

Workout #25

20 min. cardiovascular exercise at level 6 exertion

Legs

Workout #26

20 min. cardiovascular exercise at level 6 exertion

Torso

Workout #27

20 min. cardiovascular exercise at level 6 exertion

Notes:

Week 10- PHASE II Advanced Level

Goal: 3-weeks of Muscle shaping & toning employing more repititions with lighter weight. Combining big muscles

20 min. cardiovascular exercise at level 6 exertion

Chest/Back/Legs   Warmups

Exercises

Workout#28		1	2	3	4	5	6
		lb.X15-20reps	lb.X15-20reps	lb.X15-20reps	lb.X15-20reps	lb.X15-20reps	lb.X15-20reps
Set 1							
Set 2							
Set 3							

25 min. cardiovascular exercise at level 6 exertion

Shoulders/Biceps/Triceps   Warmups

Exercises

Workout#29		1	2	3	4	5	6
		lb.X15-20reps	lb.X15-20reps	lb.X15-20reps	lb.X15-20reps	lb.X15-20reps	lb.X15-20reps
Set 1							
Set 2							
Set 3							

25 min. cardiovascular exercise at level 6 exertion

Chest/Back/Legs   Warmups

Exercises

Workout#30		1	2	3	4	5	6
		lb.X15-20reps	lb.X15-20reps	lb.X15-20reps	lb.X15-20reps	lb.X15-20reps	lb.X15-20reps
Set 1							
Set 2							
Set 3							

25 min. cardiovascular exercise at level 6 exertion

Notes:

181

Week 11: Get the metabolism moving: Circuit Training

Goal: Continue to build LMT to help speed up metabolism.

Shoulders/Biceps/Triceps

25 min. cardiovascular exercise at level 6 exertion

Chest/Back/Legs

25 min. cardiovascular exercise at level 6 exertion

Shoulders/Biceps/Triceps

25 min. cardiovascular exercise at level 6 exertion

Notes:

Week 12

Notes:

Week 13- Endurance Training

Goal - 3 Weeks of endurance training with shortened rest periods. This will ensure that the metabolism stays fast.

25 min. cardiovascular exercise at level 6 exertion

30 min. cardiovascular exercise at level 6 exertion

30 min. cardiovascular exercise at level 6 exertion

Notes:

Notes

Week 15

One more week of lactic acid endurance training and then into the POWER Strength Training.

30 min. cardiovascular exercise at level 6 exertion

30 min. cardiovascular exercise at level 6 exertion

30 min. cardiovascular exercise at level 6 exertion

30 min. cardiovascular exercise at level 6 exertion

Notes:

Week 16-Power Strength Training

Goal: 3 weeks of strength training focusing on muscle growth. Remember, the more muscle you have, the more fat you will burn.

Women, don't be worried. You will not look like Zena, the muscle chick!

Notes:

Week 17

Goal: 2nd week of strength training focusing on muscle growth. Remember, the more muscle you have, the more fat you will burn.

20 min. cardiovascular exercise at level 7 exertion

Legs

Warmups

Hamstrings	Hip flexor	lower back

Exercises

	1	2	3	4	5
	lb.X6-8 reps	lb.X6-8 reps	lb.X6-8 reps	lb.X6-8 reps	lb.X12-15reps

Workout#49

Set 1					
Set 2					
Set 3					

20 min. cardiovascular exercise at level 8 exertion

Torso

Warmups

Triceps & shoulder static stretch	Static Glute Stretch

Exercises

1	2	3	4	5	6
lb.X6-8 reps	lb.X3-5 reps	lb.X6-10reps	lb.X6-10reps	lb.X6-10reps	lb.X12-15reps

Workout#50

Set 1					
Set 2					
Set 3					

20 min. cardiovascular exercise at level 8 exertion

Legs

Warmups

Hamstrings	Hip flexor	lower back

Exercises

	1	2	3	4	5
	lb.X6-8 reps	lb.X6-8 reps	lb.X6-8 reps	lb.X6-8 reps	lb.X12-15reps

Workout#51

Set 1					
Set 2					
Set 3					

Notes:

Notes:

Chapter XXI

Maintain your success

Congratulations! How does it feel? You've proven your commitment to your health and fitness and are now enjoying the benefits. Does it feel better or worse to have more muscle tone?

Do you like carrying more body fat or less? How does it feel to have energy and stamina throughout the day? Do you enjoy fitting into clothes that were too tight only eighteen weeks ago? Do you have any desire to go back to your previous unhealthy lifestyle with less muscle tone, more body fat and fewer health benefits?

I believe every person has it within his- or herself to dramatically transform their lives and improve their health and fitness. I never question a person's ability; I only question their commitment. If you've made it to this page in the book, you've demonstrated your commitment.

You may be asking yourself, "What do I do now that I have completed the eighteen weeks?" The answer is to continue your healthy lifestyle and *repeat* The Promise Fat Loss and Fitness System. You know how this system works—I want you to do it again. I want you to repeat the workouts from week one to week eighteen. However, the second time through, I want you to increase the intensity of your workouts by increasing the weights. As I mentioned previously, your body needs new stimuli in order to develop and maintain lean muscle tone. Now that you've developed strength and lean muscle tone, you need to increase the challenge to your body. Increasing weights during the workout will meet this need.

Only use weights within your capabilities. Don't risk injury by using weights that are *too* heavy. If you have any questions on how much weight to use for various exercises, please contact a personal fitness professional.

I have used this eighteen-week program with my clients for years while maintaining and developing lean muscle tissue. The program doesn't stagnate because it changes virtually every workout. I'm able to continue to stimulate clients' lean muscle tissue because I increase weights as they develop strength.

You can use the eighteen-week workout indefinitely provided you keep challenging your lean muscle tissue with increased weights. If you feel a need to do a completely different workout routine, you can visit our website, www.AlessiFit.com, or order different workouts from the order sheet located at the end of this book.

Now that you have lowered your body fat, you may either want to lower it further or maintain your current level. In order to do this, you will need to continue to weight train, eat supportive meals and perform moderate cardiovascular training. By now, you know that a supportive meal is a lean protein, a slow-releasing carbohydrate and a vegetable. Your meal frequency should still be every three to three and a half hours with serving sizes as large as your clenched fist. You'll need to continue to eat in this manner six days a week. The seventh day should still be your cheat day; enjoy yourself and eat whatever you want, in moderation.

Now that you have begun to feel the positive benefits of a healthier, fit lifestyle, I know you'll want to keep it up. You've come so far and you should be proud of yourself. As I say to my clients, "If you aren't careful, you might actually feel better and live longer!" I hope you also feel better and live longer. Good luck!

Glossary

Adipose: Body fat.

Aerobic: Means "with oxygen." Occurs during low intensity exercise like walking. In this system, it is important to perform in moderation.

Alcohol: Any intoxicating liquor.

Amino acid: A group of compounds that are the building blocks of protein and muscle.

Anaerobic: Means "without oxygen." Occurs in high-intensity activities like sprinting or weight lifting. Anaerobic exercise and developing muscle tissue is the best and quickest way to increase metabolism and reduce body fat.

Atrophy: A wasting away, or decrease in the size of muscle tissue, usually from lack of use. Atrophy can occur as quickly as forty-eight hours post-workout.

Blood sugar (glucose): Sugar in the blood, usually formed from carbohydrates.

Body fat: The accumulation of adipose tissue. Body fat is usually measured in a percentage and varies according to age and gender. One of the goals of this system is to help reduce body fat.

Burning (calories): The rate at which your body utilizes fuel, either muscle, fat or glycogen.

Calories: The amount of heat required to raise one kilogram of water one degree Celsius.

Cannibalization: The detrimental effect of breaking down lean muscle tissue to get energy or essential fatty acids.

Carbohydrate: A macronutrient composed of carbon, hydrogen and oxygen. An effective fuel source for the body. Includes starches, sugars and fibers. One gram of carbohydrates equals four calories.

Cardiovascular diseases: Diseases of the heart and blood vessels.

Cardiovascular training: A type of aerobic training that is of low intensity and long duration.

Cheat day: The one day per week you can eat whatever you like, in moderation.

Circuit training: A method of resistance training that employs the use of multiple exercises performed one after another. Usually utilizes moderately lighter weight with more repetitions.

Complex carbohydrate (polysaccharides): Composed of many monosaccharides (simple sugars). Complex carbohydrates provide energy for the body and brain. They have a higher thermal effect than simple carbohydrates.

Craving: Extreme desire, mostly from sugar or fat products.

Diabetes: A metabolism disease in which carbohydrate use is reduced and lipid and protein use is enhanced; caused by deficiency or lack of insulin. The body no longer effectively regulates blood sugar.

Diet: Short-term nutritional pattern in which calories are reduced. Not an effective way to lose fat.

Diet drugs: Both over-the-counter and prescription drugs designed to make you feel satiated (full). Over time, these drugs condition the metabolism to work slower when muscle tissue is decreased.

Endurance training: Done to sustain energy over a period of time. It is usually anaerobic such as weight lifting or sprinting.

Essential fatty acids: Fats the body cannot make, which must be obtained from food. These fats are important to cellular synthesis and hormone production. Flaxseed oil, hemp oil, fish oil and safflower oil are good sources of these fats.

Fast-releasing carbohydrate: Carbohydrates or sugars that increase blood sugar quickly. This rise is usually followed by a surge in insulin secretion. Examples include mono- and disaccharides such as fruit (fructose) and table sugar (sucrose).

Fat: One of the macronutrients, some of which are essential to carry out body processes. There are two types of fats, saturated (bad) and unsaturated (good).

Fat blockers: Prescription and over-the-counter medicine claiming to block saturated dietary fat from being stored in the body as body fat. These products will not work.

Fat oxidation: Reduction or burning of body fat.

Food manufacturers: Companies that make food products to sell in the marketplace.

Glucagon: A hormone secreted from the islets of Langerhans in the pancreas; acts primarily on the liver to release glucose into the blood. Also aids in the burning of fat.

Glycogen: A sugar formed from glucose that is stored in the muscle. These stores are used for energy and, when the stores are full, the muscles look and feel hard.

Hydration: Proper intake of water for cells of the body to be healthy.

Hydrogenated: A fat that is solid at room temperature. These fats include margarine and peanut butter, and should be limited.

Hypertension: High blood pressure.

Insulin: A hormone secreted by the pancreas that increases the uptake of glucose and amino acids by most tissues.

Labeling laws: Laws that stipulate the information that food manufacturers must include on the labels of their products. These laws have loopholes that food manufacturers can manipulate, for example, serving size.

Lipid: Usually refers to fats.

Low calorie diet: Short-term nutritional plan that is designed to limit calories so that scale weight (mostly water) can be reduced. These diets often have a negative impact on metabolism.

Macronutrient: Groups of foods that include proteins, carbohydrates and fats. Chemicals taken into the body that are used to produce energy, provide building blocks for new molecules or function in other chemical reactions.

Meal replacement shakes: Engineered foods that contain carbohydrates, protein and fats in liquid form.

Metabolism: The rate or speed at which the body processes food.

Misinformation: Information that is deceptive and misleading.

Mitochondria: Small rod shape or spherical structures in the muscles that are the site of heat and energy production and in which fat and calories are burned.

Moderate cardiovascular training: Performing a limited amount of aerobic training so that muscle is not broken down by the body for energy.

Muscle tissue: One of the four major tissue types, characterized by its contractile abilities.

Nourishment: Substances that are ingested and digested to maintain life and growth.

Obese: Excessively fat.

Periodization: A term personal trainers use for workout variation.

Plateau: A period of little positive change in the body while exercising. Usually has to do with lack of body fat reduction.

Post-workout: The period of time, usually up to forty minutes after the workout, when glycogen stores are depleted and muscle tissue is broken down.

Protein: Macronutrient consisting of long sequences of amino acids linked together by peptide bonds. Protein is the building block of muscle and has the highest thermal effect of any macronutrient.

Protein bars: Manufactured candy bars that claim to contain high amounts of protein and few carbohydrates and sugars.

Protein day: A nutritional approach designed to hasten the reduction of body fat. Should be done only on non-weight training days. Lean protein sources and vegetable should still be consumed.

Protein drinks: Synthetically manufactured protein, usually from whey or egg sources, designed to help repair muscle tissue after a workout.

Quick fix syndrome: Many Americans continuously jeopardize their health and fitness because they are unwilling to spend the necessary time to perform a complete program. They want quick results and often buy products that can be harmful or engage in a low calorie diet that slows their metabolism further.

Satiation: Feeling satisfied. Essential fatty acids satisfy the body's desire to consume foods rich in fat or sugar.

Saturated fats: Fatty acid in which the carbon chain contains only single bonds between carbon atoms. These are "bad" fats. Examples include cheese, butter, pork and palm oil.

Scale weight: The sum of your muscle, bone, water and fat expressed in pounds or kilograms. This number tells nothing of a person's body composition.

Serving size: The suggested amount or portion that food manufacturers indicate on the labels of their products. Many times this amount is extremely small.

Simple carbohydrate: A mono- or disaccharide. Includes glucose, fruit (fructose) and table sugar (sucrose). Tends to elevate blood sugar quickly.

Slow-releasing carbohydrate: Complex carbohydrates that don't quickly spike blood sugar levels because of the time it takes the body to chemically break down these sugars into glucose. Wheat bread, sweet potatoes and brown rice are examples.

Starch: Carbohydrates. Found in plants, are long chains of glucose molecules. Examples include bread, rice and potatoes.

Starving: Occurs when the body doesn't receive adequate fuel, as on various diets. It economizes and burns less fuel, thus the metabolism is conditioned to burn more slowly.

Strength training: Type of weight training that generally combines more weight with fewer repetitions.

Supplementation: Means "in addition to" not "instead of." Supplements can be used to enhance the results attained through proper nutrition and regular workouts.

Supportive foods: As used in this system, describes various types of foods that will help to build muscle, sustain energy and burn fat. They include lean protein sources, slow-releasing carbohydrates and vegetables.

Sweet tooth: The physical and psychological cravings that occur in response to sugary or high carbohydrate foods that cause a spike in blood sugar. The body releases insulin to stabilize the blood sugar level, which often dips below the normal range. The body then craves more sugar to elevate the levels to normal.

Synergy: A term used in this system to demonstrate how the combined effect of developing lean muscle tissue, eating supportive meals frequently and performing a moderate amount of cardiovascular training is greater compared to any component alone.

Thermal effect of food: The calories or energy required to process and burn food. Protein has the highest effect, carbohydrates are in the middle and fat has the lowest thermal effect.

Transform: A way to dramatically change a person's health and fitness.

Type two diabetes (mellitus): Also referred to as adult onset. Metabolic disease in which carbohydrate use is reduced and that of lipid and protein is enhanced; caused by deficiency of insulin.

Unsaturated fats: Monounsaturated includes olive and peanut oils while polyunsaturated includes flax, safflower and fish oils. These are "good" fats.

Variation: Refers to constantly changing workouts (periodization) for ongoing progress.

Weight-training (resistance): The use of free weights, body weight or machines to create force on muscle tissue. This is the most effective way to develop lean muscle tissue, increase metabolism and reduce body fat.

Sources of Information

1. American Diabetes Association. 1999 Annual Report.

2. American Heart Association. "Fiber, Lipid, and Coronary Heart Disease." *A Statement for Health Care Professionals From the Nutrition Committee*, American Heart Association, 1997.

3. Boyles, S. *WebMD Medical News.* "Looking for the Fountain of Youth? Try the Gym." September 2001.

4. Bouchard, Claude. *Physical Activity and Obesity.* Baton Rouge: Human Kinetics Publishing Inc., 2000.

5. Centers for Disease Control and Prevention. "Obesity and Overweight: A Public Health Epidemic." Online media. September, 2001.

6. Centers for Disease Control and Prevention. "Prevalence of Healthy Lifestyle Characteristics-Michigan, 1998-2000." Online media. September 2001.

7. Cigolini, M., G. Targher, A.I.A. Bergamo, M. Tonoli, F. Filippi, M. Muggeo, and G. De Sandre. "Moderate alcohol consumption and its relation to visceral fat and plasma androgens in healthy women." *International Journal of Obesity* 20:206–212, 1996.

8. Colino, S. *Self.com.* "Eat Well: The Health Payoffs of Mini Meals." March 2001.

9. Foreyt, J.P. and K. Goodrick. "The ultimate triumph of obesity." *The Lancet* 346: 134–135, 1995.

10. Forte, J. "Vegetarians Versus Meat Eaters." *Personal Fitness Professional*, September 2001.

11. *Health.com.* "Squeeze in Fitness." September 2001.

12. Kaplan, P. *The Answer.* "Personal Development." 1999.

13. Karas, J. *Business Plan for the Body.* New York: Three Rivers Press, 2001.

14. Kuzemchak, S. *Shape Magazine.* "Small Changes, Big Payoffs." April 2001.

197

15. Mayo Clinic. "Obesity." May 2001.

16. *Men's Fitness.* "23 Essential Tips for Gaining Muscle." May 2001.

17. O'Shea, M. *Parade Magazine.* "Better Fitness." September 16, 2001.

18. Philips, B. *Body for Life.* New York: Harper Collins, 1999.

19. Ryttig K.R., G. Tellnes, L. Haegh, E. Boe, H. Fagerthun. "A dietary fiber supplement and weight maintenance after weight reduction: a randomized, double blind, placebo controlled long-term trial." *International Journal of Obesity* 13:165–171, 1989.

20. Stunkard, A., Wadden T. *Obesity: Theory and Therapy.* New York: Raven Press, 1993.

21. Tremblay, A., E. Wouters, M. Wenker, S. St-Pierre, C. Bouchard, and J.P. Despres. "Alcohol and high fat diet: a combination favoring overfeeding." *American Journal of Clinical Nutrition* 62:639–644, 1995.

22. Vitetta-Miller, R. *Shape Magazine.* "Eggs For Dinner." March 2001.

23. Vitetta-Miller, R. *Shape Magazine.* "Rise and Dine." May 2001.

24. Whitaker, R.C., J.A. Wright, M.S. Pepe, K.D. Seidel, and W.H. Dietz. "Predicting obesity in young adulthood from childhood and parental obesity." *New England Journal of Medicine* 337:869–873, 1997.

25. www.ArtToday.com. Stock art.

Order Form

Please send me the following:

❏ *The Promise Fat Loss & Fitness System* Book $29.95

❏ *The Promise Fat Loss & Fitness System* audio CD $19.95

Name: _____

Address: _____

City, State, Zip: _____

Telephone: _____

E-mail address: _____

Sales tax: Please add 8% for New York residents

Shipping by air:
US: $5 for the first book or disk and $2 for each additional product.
International: $10 for first book or disk and $6 for each additional product

Payment: ❏ Visa ❏ MasterCard ❏ American Express
❏ Discover

Card number: _____

Name on card: _____ Exp. Date: _____

Card holder signature: _____

- -

- **Interactive e-mail service for The Promise**

Go to www.AlessiFit.com to find out how you can become a client of the Alessi brothers no matter where you live! Interact with Derek & Don Alessi for all of your fitness and nutrition needs. The interactive e-mail service allows you to ask questions directly to the fitness experts with regards to your personal goals.

- **Interactive e-mail service for personal trainers**

Personal Trainers can now utilize the Alessi brothers' knowledge and experience to help your own business flourish. The Alessi's have been mentoring elite-level trainers for years and now you too can share their wisdom and learn how to get astonishing results with your clients. This is an essential tool in becoming the most in-demand trainer in your area. Go to www.AlessiFit.com for details.

Order Form

📠 **Fax orders:** (716) 633-2030. Fax this form.

💻 **E-mail orders:** ThePromise@adelphia.net

   Website: www.AlessiFit.com

✉ **Mail orders:**   **Alessi Fitness**
                       7662 Transit Road
                       Williamsville, NY 14221 USA

Please send me the following:

❏ *The Promise Fat Loss & Fitness System* Book $29.95

❏ *The Promise Fat Loss & Fitness System* audio CD $19.95

Name: _____

Address: _____

City, State, Zip: _____

Telephone: _____

E-mail address: _____

Sales tax: Please add 8% for New York residents

Shipping by air:
   US: $5 for the first book or disk and $2 for each additional product.
   International: $10 for first book or disk and $6 for each additional product

Payment: ❏ Visa   ❏ MasterCard   ❏ American Express
                 ❏ Discover

Card number: _____

Name on card: _____ Exp. Date: _____

Card holder signature: _____

- -

- **Interactive e-mail service for The Promise**

Go to www.AlessiFit.com to find out how you can become a client of the Alessi brothers no matter where you live! Interact with Derek & Don Alessi for all of your fitness and nutrition needs. The interactive e-mail service allows you to ask questions directly to the fitness experts with regards to your personal goals.

- **Interactive e-mail service for personal trainers**

Personal Trainers can now utilize the Alessi brothers' knowledge and experience to help your own business flourish. The Alessi's have been mentoring elite-level trainers for years and now you too can share their wisdom and learn how to get astonishing results with your clients. This is an essential tool in becoming the most in-demand trainer in your area. Go to www.AlessiFit.com for details.

Order Form

Fax orders: (716) 633-2030. Fax this form.

E-mail orders: ThePromise@adelphia.net

Website: www.AlessiFit.com

Mail orders:
    Alessi Fitness
    7662 Transit Road
    Williamsville, NY 14221 USA

Please send me the following:

❏ *The Promise Fat Loss & Fitness System* Book $29.95

❏ *The Promise Fat Loss & Fitness System* audio CD $19.95

Name: _____

Address: _____

City, State, Zip: _____

Telephone: _____

E-mail address: _____

Sales tax: Please add 8% for New York residents

Shipping by air:
    US: $5 for the first book or disk and $2 for each additional product.
    International: $10 for first book or disk and $6 for each additional product

Payment: ❏ Visa   ❏ MasterCard   ❏ American Express   ❏ Discover

Card number: _____

Name on card: _____ Exp. Date: _____

Card holder signature: _____

- -

- **Interactive e-mail service for The Promise**

Go to www.AlessiFit.com to find out how you can become a client of the Alessi brothers no matter where you live! Interact with Derek & Don Alessi for all of your fitness and nutrition needs. The interactive e-mail service allows you to ask questions directly to the fitness experts with regards to your personal goals.

- **Interactive e-mail service for personal trainers**

Personal Trainers can now utilize the Alessi brothers' knowledge and experience to help your own business flourish. The Alessi's have been mentoring elite-level trainers for years and now you too can share their wisdom and learn how to get astonishing results with your clients. This is an essential tool in becoming the most in-demand trainer in your area. Go to www.AlessiFit.com for details.